The New 21-Day High Fat Low Carb Diet Plan 2021

Easy Low Carb Recipes

CONTENTS

INTRODUCTION
Low Carb Diet and Its Principles

The low-carb, high-fat eating plan, or LCHF diet, is promoted as a healthy and safe way to lose weight.

The Low Carb High Fat diet uses foods high in fat and proteins. In this case, carbohydrates (carbs) should be excluded entirely from the «keto» diet or reduced to a minimum in LCHF.

Originally, the Low Carb diet was developed for people with epilepsy and obesity. Now, it is actively used among athletes who want to tone their bodies to perfection. Women who dream of a more refined figure without having to do many physical exercises use the high fat low carb diet.

On a low carb diet, fat becomes the body's primary source of energy. This diet can include any fat, but carbohydrates should be reduced to zero. Carbohydrates enter the body and get processed into glucose, and glucose is very important for brain function and is the brain's primary fuel. Once there are no carbohydrates, and glucose, the body will start looking for an alternative source of fuel. This is fat, which is converted into fatty acids and ketone bodies.

Ketone bodies are a separate group of metabolic products. They are formed in the liver. Main types are acetone, acetoacetic acid, and beta-oxybutyric acid. In the ketogenic diet and the HFLC diet, ketone bodies are the primary source of energy for the brain. When doing a keto diet, the body itself enters a special state: ketosis. In ketosis, the body is tuned to split fat to obtain ketone bodies constantly. So the person that is doing a high fat and low carbs diet actively consumes fat, but also actively loses it by feeding energy to the brain.

Low Carb vs Ketogenic Diet

What are the differences?

TYPE OF FOOD	LOW CARB	KETO
HIGH-FAT DAIRY (BUTTER, CREAM, CHEESE)	✓	✓
MILK/YOGURT	✓	MODERATION
FRUIT IN GENERAL	MODERATION	X
LOW-SUGAR FRUIT (BERRIES, OLIVES, AVOCADO)	✓	MODERATION
FISH	✓	✓
MEAT	✓	✓
LEAFY GREEN VEGETABLES	✓	✓
NUTS	✓	MODERATION
ROOT VEGETABLES	X	MODERATION
LEGUMES	MODERATION	✓
CANDY	X	X
DARK CHOCOLATE (IDEALLY 80% +)	✓	MODERATION
GRAINS, BREAD, AND GRAIN PRODUCTS	X	X
CRUCIFEROUS/GREEN VEGETABLES	✓	X

The most notable difference between the ketogenic diet and LCHF diets is that the ketogenic diet has a strict limit on carbohydrates, while LCHF does not.

Who Is Suitable for HFLC Diet?

The ketogenic diet is effective for rapid weight loss when you need to lose extra pounds in a short period of time. Such a diet can easily control appetite and let you forget about being hungry for a long time.

This diet is not suitable for people

- with gastrointestinal disease,
- any type of diabetes,
- liver and kidney disease,
- during pregnancy and lactation,
- when working in harsh and dangerous conditions,
- for people that do mentally demanding jobs.

In addition, athletes that want to gain muscle mass should not use it.

Before starting the ketogenic diet, it is absolutely necessary to consult with a doctor, as he/she will determine whether this diet suits you and your body.

Pros and Cons for Anyone Going Low-Carb High-Fat Diet

The most important advantage of a ketogenic diet is that it gives the ability to shed an impressive amount of excess weight in a very short time. For example, it is quite possible to lose 20 pounds in just 2 weeks! In this case, a person loses only fat, whereas muscle mass remains.

Simple Rules for the Low Carb Diet

Our HFLC meal plan contains a lot of useful information that will help you begin the process of dieting. We made a menu for 21 days, and every one of 100 dishes have nutritional information.

For you to properly start the low carb diet and achieve results, you must follow the following recommendations:

- during the 1st week, the daily menu will have up to 40 grams of carbs per day to make it easier for you to start the diet; also in the 1st week you will be getting up to 40% of calories from carbohydrates;

- during the 2nd and 3d weeks, the daily menu will have up to 30 grams of carbs per day;
- during the low-calorie day avoid doing active sports.

<u>Some useful keto friendly ideas:</u>

- Get a lot of your calories from fat, a moderate amount from protein, and very few from carbs.
- Fat: 70% of calories/ Protein: 25% of calories/ Carbs: 5% of calories.
- Do not use «carbs» food, except for vegetables and avocados.
- Eat fatty meat.
- Add cheese, salad dressing, nuts, if you need to add a bit more into each meal to make sure you are reaching your goals.

WEEK 1

MEAL	Breakfast	Lunch	Snacks	Dinner	Dessert
			Week 1		
SUNDAY	Cheddar Taco Crisps	Greek Salad	Avocado Chicken Roll	Venison Spring Keto Stew	Nuts' Keto Sweets and Peanut-Cream
MONDAY	Keto Cobb Salad	Savory Bacon Cranberry Cheese Tartlets	Marinated Olive with Cheese	Burgundy Beef Stew	Carrot Nut Cake
TUESDAY	Fried Kale with Pork and Cranberries	Buffalo Deviled Eggs	Keto Pizza	Roasted Turkey with Rosemary Thyme Gravy	Lemon and Blackberry Pudding
WEDNESDAY	Creamy Mashed Potatoes with Cauliflower	Creamy Low Carb Butternut Squash Soup	Pig Tongue	Turkey Rolls and Vegetables	Coconut Snowballs
THURSDAY	Horseradish, Caramelized Onion and	Bacon and Eggs	Celery Root with Mushrooms and Gorgonzola	Keto Turkey Stew	Nuts' Keto Sweets and Peanut-Cream
FRIDAY	Celery Crunch Salad	Bok Choy Soup	Dried Chicken Breast a la "Carpaccio"	Stuffed Pork Tenderloin Wrapped in Bacon	Coconut Snowballs
SATURDAY	Avocado and Chicken Salad with Bacon	Cauliflower Cream Soup	Buffalo Chicken Meatballs	Beef Stew	Vegan Chocolate Turron

WEEK 1 SHOPPING LIST

PANTRY STAPLES	VEGETABLES
Butter	Avocados – 2 total
Butternut squash	Blackberries - ½ cup
Tuna – 8 cans	Cranberries frozen – 12 oz
Campari tomatoes – 3 lb	Onions – 8 total
Almond flour - ½ lb	Celery - 1 package
Coconut flour – ½ cup	Kale – 1 lb
Coconut Milk – 2 pack	Lemon – 4 total
	Cauliflower -2 lb
DAIRY & MEAT	Carrots – 7 total
Sour Cream – 1 container (16 oz)	Spinach – 2 oz
Soft Cream Cheese – 3 containers	Broccoli – 8 oz frozen
Cheddar Cheese – 8 oz	Bok choy – 2 cup
Eggs – 36 total	Olives – 4 oz
Bacon slices – 40 oz	
Blue Cheese – 1 cup	**OTHER**
Chicken – 2 lb	Agave Syrup
Chicken breast – 3 lb	Hazelnuts – 4 oz
Gorgonzola cheese – 6 oz	Mushrooms - 12 oz
Ground pork – 1 lb	Pecans – 10 oz
Mozzarella – 16 oz	
Stew meat – 3 lb	
Turkey – 5 lb	
Pork tenderloin -1 lb	
Parmesan cheese grated – 3 oz	
Pig tongue – 4 lb	
Beef snack, tail – 5 lb	
Beef Stew – 2 lb	

DAY 1

Cheddar Taco Crisps
Greek Salad
Avocado Chicken Roll
Venison Spring Keto Stew
Nuts Keto Sweets and Peanut-Cream

Fat - 101g   Carbs - 34g   Protein -84g   Calories -1364

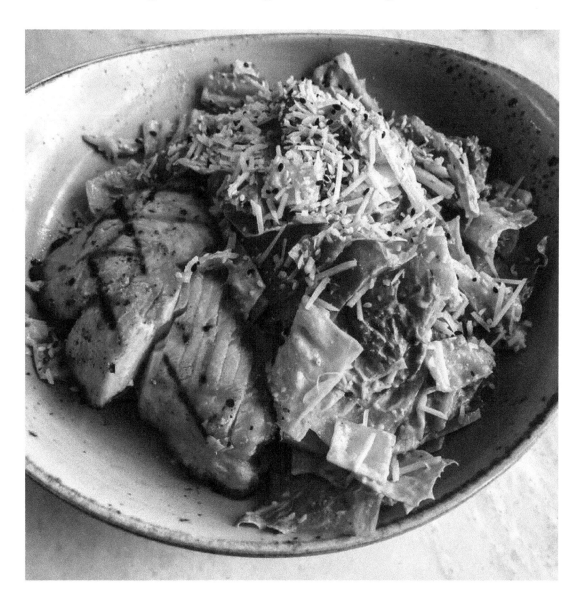

CHEDDAR TACO CRISPS

6 serves | 15 min

Ingredients

¾ cup full-fat cheddar, finely shredded

¼ cup parmesan, shredded

¼ teaspoon chili powder

¼ teaspoon ground cumin

Large pinch of cayenne pepper

Directions

1. Preheat oven to 400°F.
2. Line a baking sheet with a silicone baking mat.
3. Mix the Cheddar, Parmesan, chili powder, cumin, and cayenne in a small bowl.
4. Place heaping tablespoonful's of the cheese mixture on the baking sheet 1 inch apart.
5. Spread out each pile, and pat down lightly.
6. Cook about 5 min. Bake until the cheese is golden brown and bubbly.
7. Let the crisps cool for a few seconds on the baking sheet.
8. Using a metal spatula, lift and drape the crisps over a rolling pin to cool completely.
9. Eat or store in an airtight container at room temperature for about 2 days.

Fat - 7g   Carbs - 1g   Protein -7g Calories -88

GREEK SALAD
4 serves | 15 min

Ingredients

2 ripe tomatoes

½ cucumber

½ red onion

½ green bell pepper

7 ounces Feta cheese

10 lack olives

2 tablespoons olive oil

½ tablespoon red wine vinegar

2 teaspoons dried oregano

salt and pepper

Directions

Salad

1. Cut the tomatoes and cucumber into bite-sized pieces.
2. Thinly slice the bell pepper and onion.
3. Arrange the ingredients on a plate.
4. Add feta and olives.
5. Drizzle the salad with the dressing.
6. Sprinkle with oregano.

<u>Dressing</u>

Mix the olive oil and vinegar. Add salt and pepper to taste.

Fat - 20g Carbs - 10g Protein -9g Calories -252

AVOCADO CHICKEN ROLL

1 serves | 15 min

Ingredients

4 ounces fried chicken breast

1 tablespoon mayonnaise

½ medium avocado

salt

pepper

Directions

1. Cut the chicken into thin long strips.
2. Cut avocado into medium slices, put them in a plate, mix with mayonnaise and salt and pepper to taste.
3. Put avocado mixture on the meat strips. Roll strips.

Fat - 29g   Carbs - 13g   Protein -36g   Calories -450

VENISON SPRING KETO STEW

4 serves | 4 h 20 min

Ingredients

1 pound venison

2 tablespoons olive oil

1 bulb garlic

1 cup shredded cabbage (purple)

1 cup sliced celery

4 cups bone broth

1 teaspoon salt

1 teaspoon pepper

2 cups chopped asparagus

2 bay leaves

Directions

1. At first, peel and slice garlic. Cut it into 1/8-inch thin slices.
2. Slice the purple cabbage.
3. Slice celery.
4. Preheat the skillet. Pour olive oil in it.
5. Add celery, garlic, bay leaves to the skillet. Saute the ingredients for about 5-6 minutes until tender.
6. Add venison to the cabbage. Salt and pepper. Cook until the meat is brown.
7. Take a big saucepan. Place cabbage and venison in it, add broth.
8. Stew for 4 hours. Add water if the stew is dry.
9. When done, add chopped asparagus in the saucepan.
10. Serve the stew with olive oil and lime.

Fat - 16g   Carbs - 8g   Protein -32g   Calories-310

NUTS' KETO SWEETS AND PEANUT-CREAM

4 serves | 2 h 15 min

Ingredients

½ cup coconut oil

1 tablespoon cocoa powder

½ teaspoon sweetener

vanilla

almonds, walnuts, peanuts, and/or hazelnuts

peanut paste to taste

butter to taste

Directions

1. Prepare a water bath. Melt coconut oil, but do not overheat.
2. Add cocoa and sweetener to melted oil. Add vanilla to taste. Stir. You can change the number of ingredients if you want. Pour half the contents into molds.
3. Put the nut or peanut-cream filling in each candy. Cover with rest of coconut oil mixture and sprinkle cocoa powder on the sweets with nuts immediately. Place in the refrigerator to harden.
4. Wait for the bottom layer of the candy to cool before stuffing. Mix ¼ pound of paste and 1 ounce of oil (or your choice). Add to the thickened bottom layer of chocolates. Then cover with the second part of the mixture.
5. Put the candy in the fridge. Keep the keto-candies in the cold.

Fat - 29g   Carbs – 2,4g   Protein -1g   Calories -264

DAY 2

Keto Cobb Salad
Savory Bacon Cranberry Cheese Tartlets
Marinated Olive with Cheese
Burgundy Beef Stew
Carrot Nut Cake

Fat – 144 g   Carbs - 37g   Protein -75g   Calories -1543

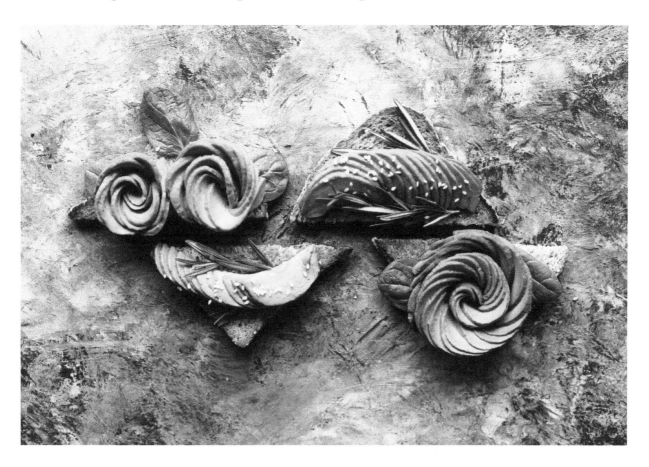

KETO COBB SALAD

4 serves | 20 min

Ingredients

2 cherry tomatoes

½ avocado

1 hard-boiled egg

2 cups mixed green salad

 2 ounces cooked chicken breast

1 ounce feta cheese

¼ cup cooked bacon

1 tablespoon olive oil

½ tablespoon white wine vinegar

Salt and pepper

Directions

1. Cut the tomatoes, egg, and avocadoes into slices.
2. Shred cooked chicken breast.
3. Crumble feta cheese.
4. Place the mixed green salad into salad bowl or on a plate.
5. Place tomatoes, avocado, egg, bacon, cheese, and chicken on top of the salad.

Dress the salad with olive oil and white wine vinegar. Salt and pepper to taste. You can use one tablespoon Ranch dressing.

Fat - 15g   Carbs – 7g   Protein -10g   Calories -190

SAVORY BACON CRANBERRY CHEESE TARTLETS

6 serves | 1 h

Ingredients

<u>Tart crust</u>

1 cups blanched almond flour

1 egg

1/5 cup butter melted

⅛ teaspoon sea salt

<u>Filling</u>

3 chopped bacon slices

½ cups cubed Mahon Menorca Semi-Cured cheese

1/4 cup unsweetened dried cranberries

1 teaspoon fresh thyme leaves

salt

black pepper to taste

Directions

1. Preheat oven to 370 °F. Grease 6-cup muffin pan.
2. Combine the ingredients for the crust. Form dough.
3. Make 6 balls with your hands. Place one into each cup.
4. Press dough with a small glass to make the tart crusts.
5. Bake the crusts for 7 minutes until lightly golden. Remove them from the oven.
6. Fill the crusts with fried and chopped bacon, cubed Mahon Menorca cheese, and dried cranberries.
7. Sprinkle the tartlets with salt, pepper, and fresh thyme leaves.
8. Bake for 10 minutes or until cheese is completely melted.
9. Remove the tartlets and cool for 10 minutes.

Fat - 26g Carbs – 8g   Protein -19g   Calories -158

MARINATED OLIVE WITH CHEESE

8 serves | 8 h 30 min

Ingredients

4 ounces cream cheese, cold

5 ounces sharp white cheddar cheese

1/6 cup pimiento-stuffed olives

1/6 cup pitted greek olives

1/8 cup balsamic vinegar

1/8 cup olive oil

1 teaspoon fresh parsley, minced

1 teaspoon fresh basil, minced

1 garlic cloves, minced

1 ounce canned pimiento strips, drained and chopped

Directions

1. Cut the cheese in half lengthwise. Cut each half into 1/4-inch slices.
2. Arrange cheeses upright in a ring on a serving plate. Alternate cheddar and cream cheese slices.
3. Place olives in the center of the plate.
4. Whisk vinegar, oil, parsley, basil, and garlic in a small bowl until blended.
5. Drizzle the seasoning over olives and cheese.
6. Sprinkle the ingredients with the pimientos.
7. Cool at least 8 hours or overnight in the refrigerator.

Fat - 16g   Carbs – 2g   Protein -6g   Calories -168

BURGUNDY BEEF STEW

6 serves | 2 h 10 min

Ingredients

2 teaspoons avocado oil

2 pounds beef stew chunks

2 bacon slices

4 cups bone broth

2 small carrots

4 ounces green beans

¼ medium onion

2 tablespoons cumin powder

1 tablespoon turmeric

1 tablespoon garlic powder

1 teaspoon ginger powder

Salt and pepper to taste

Directions

1. Peel and chop the carrots, onion, beans.
2. Chop beef chunks into small pieces.
3. Dice bacon slices.
4. Take a large pot and pour olive oil in it. Brown the beef stew chunks in the oil over high heat.
5. Add vegetables, spices to the beef. Cover the pot; simmer the stew on medium heat for 90 min. Stir occasionally.
6. Season stew with salt and pepper.
7. Meanwhile, take a small skillet. Preheat it. Fry bacon until crispy, for 2-3 minutes.
8. Add frying bacon to the ready stew.

Fat - 41g   *Carbs – 3g*   *Protein -27g*   *Calories -507*

CARROT NUT CAKE

4 serves | 1 h 10 min

Ingredients

2 ounces almond flour

1 ounce coconut flour

2 tablespoons baking powder

2 ounces pecan

2 tablespoons chia seeds

4 ounces grated carrot

4 chicken eggs

3 ounces philadelphia cream cheese

3 ounces sour cream (30%)

3 ounces butter

vanilla, cinnamon, salt

Directions

1. Preheat oven to 320 ºF.
2. Prepare the cream. In a blender, place the cream cheese, sour cream and vanilla to taste. Mix everything well until smooth. Allow the mixture to sit.
3. Mix almond and coconut flour, chia seeds and pecans. Add baking powder, salt, and cinnamon. Grind all these dry ingredients in the flour. You can leave large pieces.
4. Grated carrot.
5. Separate the yolks in the eggs. Beat the eggs white to add air. Mix the yolks.
6. Melt the butter and let cool. Mix the egg whites with the yolks. Add creamy melted butter. Mix again.
7. In the mixture add dry Ingredients mix flour, nuts and seeds. Gently stir manually or with a blender.
8. Fold the carrots evenly into the batter.
9. Place the batter onto a baking sheet and bake in the oven for 45 min.

10. Cool the cake and cut into several layers. Smear each layer with cream. Let the cake rest overnight in the refrigerator.

Fat - 46g   Carbs – 17g   Protein -13g   Calories -520

DAY 3

Fried Kale with Pork and Cranberries

Buffalo Deviled Eggs

Keto Pizza

Roasted Turkey with Rosemary Thyme Gravy

Lemon and Blackberry Pudding

Fat - 113g   Carbs - 40g   Protein -150g Calories -1848

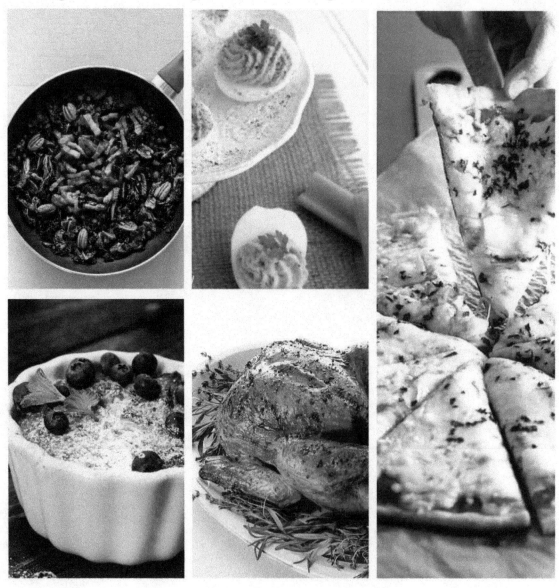

FRIED KALE WITH PORK AND CRANBERRIES

4 serves | 20 min

Ingredients

3 ounces butter
1 pound kale
2/3 pound smoked pork belly or bacon
2 ounces walnuts or pecans
½ cup frozen cranberries
Salt and black pepper to taste

Directions

1. Rinse, trim, and chop kale into large chunks. Set aside.
2. Use the strips of bacon or cut the pork into strips. Fry over medium heat until golden brown and crispy.
3. Place kale into the pan. Fry 3-5 minutes until wilted.
4. Add salt and pepper to taste. Turn off the heat.

Add cranberries and nuts to the kale and bacon or pork. Stir the ingredients.

Fat - 56g   Carbs – 17g   Protein -34g   Calories -692

BUFFALO DEVILED EGGS
6 serves | 20 min

Ingredients

6 hard boiled chicken eggs, large

½ pound boiled and chopped chicken

¼ onion

¼ cup blue cheese crumbles

¼ cup Franks Buffalo Wing Sauce

1 small chopped celery

2 tablespoons blue cheese dressing

Directions

1. Boil the eggs.
2. Chop the chicken and celery.
3. Peel cooked and cooled eggs. Cut them in half lengthwise. Separate the yolks from the egg whites and place yolks in mixing bowl.
4. Add chicken, celery, blue cheese, Franks Buffalo Wing Sauce and dressing to yolks.
5. Press the onion and add juice to the bowl. Mix all the ingredients.
6. Stuff the egg whites with yolk mixture using a fork or spoon. You can also pipe the yolks into the whites using a Ziploc bag with the tip cut off.

Fat - 18g   Carbs – 2g   Protein -19g   Calories -253

LEMON AND BLACKBERRY PUDDING

4 serves | 35 min

Ingredients

¼cup coconut flour

5 chicken eggs

2 tablespoons butter

2 tablespoons coconut oil

2 tablespoons oily cream

2 tablespoons erythritol

1 lemon

2 teaspoons lemon juice

1/2 cup blackberries

1/4 teaspoon baking powder

10 drops liquid stevia

Directions

1. Preheat oven to 345 ºF.
2. Separate egg yolks from whites. Whisk the yolks to a pale yellow color. Add erythritol and stevia and mix until evenly combined.
3. Add fatty cream, coconut oil, and lemon juice.
4. Wash and zest the lemon. Add zest to the mixture and mix.
5. Add the coconut flour and baking powder. Mix all the ingredients.
6. Add the blackberry to the mixture. Press the berries into it a little.
7. Bake pudding for 20-25 min. in the baking cups.

Fat - 14g Carbs – 16g   Protein -6g   Calories -177

KETO PIZZA

8 serves | 1 h

Ingredients

Sauce

1/3 cup canned sugar-free crushed tomatoes

1 teaspoon olive oil

1 small clove garlic, minced

A pinch of kosher salt

Keto Dough

1 ½ cups shredded mozzarella

2 tablespoons full-fat sour cream

2/3 cup almond flour

2 large eggs, lightly beaten

A pinch of kosher salt

Olive oil

Toppings

1/3 cup shredded whole-milk Mozzarella

Crushed red pepper flakes and dried oregano, for sprinkling

Directions

Sauce

1. Combine the tomatoes, minced garlic, and salt in a small bowl.
2. Let the mixture sit for 30 min. at room temperature.

Dough

1. Place the cheese and sour cream in a large microwave-safe bowl.
2. Microwave the ingredients in one-minute intervals, stirring until the cheese is melted. Cool the mixture slightly.

3. Add the eggs, flour, and ¼ teaspoon of salt to the cheese mixture. Mix with your hands until a stretchy, slightly wet dough forms.

Pizza

1. Adjust an oven rack to the low position and place a baking sheet on it.
2. Preheat oven to 450 ˚F.
3. Grease a piece of parchment paper with olive oil.
4. Lightly coat your hands in oil and place the dough on the parchment, patting into a ¼-inch-thick rectangle. Make the edges a bit thicker to create a crust all around.
5. Place the dough on the baking sheet. Bake until puffy and golden. Cook about 15 min.
6. Remove the dough from the oven and top with sauce and mozzarella. Bake pizza until it's heated through and cheese is melted, about 5 min.
7. Remove the dough from the oven.
8. Sprinkle with pepper flakes, salt, and oregano.

Fat - 5g   Carbs – 1g   Protein -4g   Calories -160

ROASTED TURKEY WITH ROSEMARY THYME GRAVY

6 serves | 4 h 30 min

Ingredients

Roasted Turkey

2 ½ pounds whole turkey

½ small onion

1 small lemon

¼ cup minced garlic

1 teaspoon dried rosemary

2 chopped stalks green onions

Turkey Coating

2 tablespoons melted butter

1 teaspoon cayenne

1 teaspoon chicken herb seasoning

Gravy

Leftover parts of turkey

1/5 cup chicken stock

1 and 1/2 cups water

1 teaspoon Worcestershire

1 stalks green onions

2 brussels sprouts

1 tablespoon bacon fat

2 sprigs fresh thyme

1 bay leaf

¼ teaspoon xanthan gum

¼ cup heavy cream

Salt and pepper

Directions

1.   Preheat oven to 325 °F. Stuff the turkey with onion, lemon, minced garlic, dried rosemary, and chopped green onions.
2.   Mix the coating ingredients. Brush the turkey with this mixture.
3.   Bake turkey for 150 minutes.
4.   Boil the turkey innards in water and chicken broth for 1 hour.
5.   Add brussels sprouts. Green onion, Worcestershire, salt, and pepper to the gravy. Boil for 30-45 minutes. Then blend gravy.
6.   Add sprigs of fresh thyme, bay leaf, and heavy cream. Bring to a rolling boil.
7.   Stir Continuously. Let gravy reduce for 15-20 minutes. It should be relatively thick. Add the xanthan gum, and mix well.

Let turkey rest. Serve with gravy.

Fat - 20g   Carbs – 3g   Protein -88g   Calories -566

DAY 4

Creamy Mashed Potatoes with Cauliflower
Creamy Low Carb Butternut Squash Soup
Pig Tongue
Turkey Rolls and Vegetables
Coconut Snowballs
Fat - 120g   Carbs - 43g   Protein -95g   Calories -1680

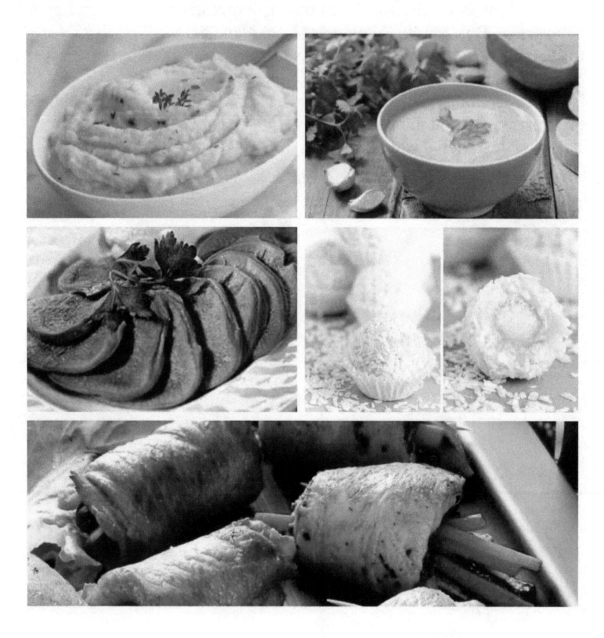

CREAMY MASHED POTATOES WITH CAULIFLOWER

3 serves | 30 min

Ingredients

2/3 pound riced cauliflower

½ cup sour cream

3 tablespoons heavy whipping cream

3 tablespoons butter

¼ tablespoon garlic powder

4 tablespoons Parmesan cheese

2 tablespoons chopped chives

Salt and pepper

Directions

1. Place the cauliflower on a deep plate, and cover with paper towel. Microwave cauliflower for 5 minutes. You can roast or steam it too. Cauliflower must be slightly soft.
2. Add sour cream, heavy whipping cream, butter, garlic powder, Parmesan cheese, salt, pepper to taste. Mix the ingredients with an immersion blender.
3. Add 1 tablespoon of chopped chives to the mixture. Mix well.
4. You can serve the dish with mashed potatoes and 1 tablespoon chives.

Fat - 28g   Carbs – 8g   Protein -7g   Calories -300

CREAMY LOW CARB BUTTERNUT SQUASH SOUP

8 serves | 1 h 10 min

Ingredients

2 pounds butternut squash, cut in half without seeds

2 tablespoons avocado oil

sea salt

black pepper

2 minced cloves of garlic

2 tablespoons fresh thyme

½ teaspoon cinnamon

1/8 teaspoon nutmeg

4 cups chicken bone broth (or broth to your taste)

1 ½ cup coconut milk

Directions

1. Preheat the oven to 400 °F. Line a baking sheet with parchment paper. Place the butternut squash halves open side up on the baking sheet.
2. Drizzle butternut squash with 1 tablespoon of avocado oil. Sprinkle with sea salt and black pepper. Flip over, face down.
3. Roast it in the oven for 40-55 minutes.
4. Take a large pot. Heat 1 tablespoon of avocado oil in it over medium heat.
5. Add minced garlic, nutmeg, thyme, cinnamon. Saute for 1 minute.
6. Add the broth, coconut milk. Cook for 20 minutes.
7. Scoop the squash. Add it into the soup. Puree until smooth with the immersion blender.
8. Saute on the low heat for 3 minutes. Serve.

Fat - 12g   Carbs – 4g   Protein -4g   Calories -183

PIG TONGUE

6 serves | 50 min

Ingredients

2 pounds pig tongue

1 stick cinnamon

2 pieces badian

5 peppercorns black pepper

2 bay leaves

1 pinch of chili pepper

1 clove garlic

1 ounce celery root

3-4 pinches of salt

For cranberry sauce

½ pound cranberries, fresh or frozen

2 teaspoons sugar

1 pinch of salt

2 teaspoons water

Directions

1. Wash the pork tongue and place in a saucepan. Cover with water, add the spices, and bring to a boil.
2. Boil on a medium heat for 35-40 min.
3. Remove from the heat. Rinse the tongue with cold water and peel.
4. Place the cranberries in saucepan. Add sugar, salt, and water.
5. Cook the ingredients on medium heat for 15 min.
6. Sieve the cranberry mass. If the sauce is too thin, reduce over low heat.
7. Cut pork tongue into thin slices, serve on a plate with cranberry sauce on top.

Fat - 47g   Carbs – 7g   Protein -61g   Calories -712

TURKEY ROLLS AND VEGETABLES

4 serves | 30 min

Ingredients

1 pound turkey breast

½ pound cream cheese

1 avocado

1 bell pepper

1 cucumber

1 tablespoon. mayonnaise

1 garlic clove

Lemon juice

salt

pepper

Directions

1. Wash and dry the turkey breast, if necessary.
2. Mix the lemon juice, chopped garlic, and pepper. Place the turkey on a deep plate. Pour lemon juice over it and leave for two hours.
3. From time to time turn the turkey to soaking well.
4. Preheat the oven to 350 ℉.
5. Place the turkey on a baking sheet. Bake for 30-40 minutes in the oven.
6. Cool the turkey.
7. Put slightly softened cream cheese into a plate. Stir with a mixer to a creamy consistency.
8. Peel the avocado. Mush with a fork, and add a couple drops of lemon juice and salt.
9. Mix avocado and cream cheese. Add a spoonful of mayo. Stir again with a mixer. You should get a thick sauce.
   Cut pepper and cucumber into thin strips.
10. Slice baked and cooled turkey. Spread cheese and avocado sauce on the turkey with.
11. Put pieces of pepper and cucumber on meat. Make small rolls.

Fat - 30g Carbs – 16g   Protein -23g   Calories -420

COCONUT SNOWBALLS

5 serves | 10 min

Ingredients

2 ounces shredded coconut

1 ounce almond flour

1 ½ ounce agave syrup

Directions

1. Mix 1 ½ ounce shredded coconut, flour, and syrup in a food processor until well combined.
2. Make 10 balls using your hands.
3. Roll the balls in ½ ounce shredded coconut.

You can keep these balls in a sealed container in a fridge for one week.

Fat - 4g   Carbs – 8g   Protein -1g   Calories -65

DAY 5

Horseradish, Caramelized Onion and Cauliflower Mash

Bacon and Eggs

Celery Root with Mushrooms and Gorgonzola

Keto Turkey Stew

Nuts' Keto Sweets and Peanut-Cream

Fat - 110g   Carbs - 31g   Protein -40g   Calories -1221

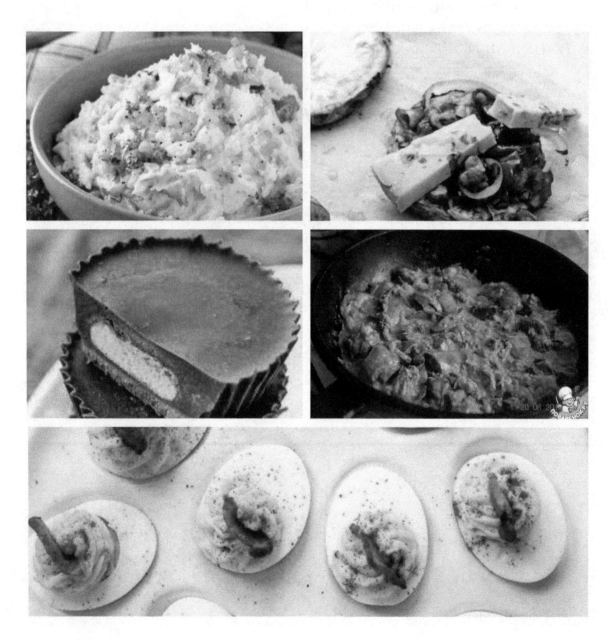

HORSERADISH, CARAMELIZED ONION AND CAULIFLOWER MASH

8 serves | 50 min

Ingredients

1 medium onion

1 large cleaned, trimmed cauliflower

2 tablespoons minced garlic

2 tablespoons olive oil

2 tablespoons butter

¼ cup sour cream

¼ cup creamy horseradish

Salt (sea) and pepper to taste

Directions

1. In a large sauté pan, place onions, garlic, olive oil, butter, salt and pepper. Cook over medium-low heat until onion caramelizes, about 30 minutes.
2. While onion caramelizes, add 4 cups water to a large sauce pan. Steam the cauliflower for 15 minutes over high heat. Then, drain the water and remove in the sauce pan.
3. Mash the cauliflower in the pan with the fork. Add caramelized onion, horseradish sauce, and sour cream to the pan. Mix all the ingredients well.

Fat - 10g Carbs – 4g   Protein -1g   Calories -147

BACON AND EGGS
10 serves | 15 min

Ingredients

5 eggs

3 tablespoons homemade mayonnaise

2 slices bacon (thick cut)

1 tablespoon pickle relish (sugar free)

Directions

1. Peel hard-boiled eggs. Cut each in half lengthwise. Fry bacon.
2. Separate the yolks from the egg whites. Crumble yolks with a fork in a large bowl.
3. Then add Mayonnaise to the yolks. Mix until the mixture looks like batter.
4. Add pickle relish. Mix all the ingredients again.
5. Cool and crumble bacon. Add it to the yolk mixture.
6. Fill the eggs' halves with the yolk. Use fork for this.
7. You can sprinkle the deviled eggs with paprika.

Fat - 5g   Carbs – 2g   Protein -4g   Calories -67

CELERY ROOT WITH MUSHROOMS AND GORGONZOLA

4 serves | 50 min

Ingredients

1 pound celery root

3 tablespoons olive oil

¼ pound mushrooms

3 ounces spinach leaves

3 ounces hazelnut

3 tablespoons butter

1 red onion, chopped

1/3 ounces Gorgonzola cheese

Salt and pepper, to taste

Directions

1. Preheat oven to 400 °F.
2. Wash and peel the celery root. Cut the root into slices or rings, 1 to 1 1/2 cm thick.
3. Smear both sides of slices with olive oil, salt, and pepper
4. Place parchment paper on the baking sheet. Put the celery on the parchment and bake in the oven for 40-45 min. until the celery becomes soft and golden.
5. Fry the mushrooms in butter until brown. Add salt and pepper.
6. Place the hazelnuts in a dry pan and fry for 5-7 min. Then, cool and chop nuts in half.
7. To make salad, mix spinach leaves, chopped red onion, mushrooms and hazelnuts in a bowl.
8. Put the salad on the cooked celery. Top with a piece of cheese and a drizzle of olive oil.

Fat - 42g Carbs – 19g   Protein -14g   Calories -428

KETO TURKEY STEW

5 serves | 5 h

Ingredients

1 pound of turkey thighs and leg meat, diced

1 clove garlic, crushed

1 tablespoon olive oil

2 ounces bacon, diced

½ teaspoon salt

½ teaspoon white ground pepper

1/3 pound button mushrooms

1/2 cup heavy cream

1 leek, halved and sliced

1 tablespoon fresh thyme leaves

1/2 teaspoons xanthan gum

1 tablespoon whole grain mustard

¼ cup parsley, roughly chopped

Directions

1.   Brown the turkey meat in the olive oil in a large non-stick frying pan over high heat. Then shift it into a slow cooker.
2.   Fry garlic, leek and bacon for 3-5 minutes until the leek has softened.
3.   Add this mixture to the meat along with thyme, salt, pepper, and mushrooms.
4.   Mix the xanthan gum, mustard, and cream. Then send it to the slow cooker, while stirring well.
5.   Cook for 2 hours on high heat.
6.   Stir through the parsley and serve alone or with a side of Creamy Broccoli Mash.

Fat - 24g Carbs – 4g   Protein -20g   Calories -315

NUTS' KETO SWEETS AND PEANUT-CREAM

4 serves | 15 min

Ingredients

½ cup coconut oil

1 tablespoon cocoa powder

½ teaspoon sweetener

vanilla

almonds, walnuts, peanuts, and/or hazelnuts

peanut paste to taste

butter to taste

Directions

1. Prepare a water bath. Melt coconut oil, but do not overheat.
2. Add cocoa and sweetener to melted oil. Add vanilla to taste. Stir. You can change the number of ingredients if you want. Pour half the contents into molds.
3. Put the nut or peanut-cream filling in each candy. Cover with rest of coconut oil mixture and sprinkle cocoa powder on the sweets with nuts immediately. Place in the refrigerator to harden.
4. Wait for the bottom layer of the candy to cool before stuffing. Mix 100 g of paste and 30 g of oil (or your choice). Add to the thickened bottom layer of chocolates. Then cover with the second part of the mixture.
5. Put the candy in the fridge. Keep the keto-candies in the cold.

Fat - 29g   Carbs – 3g   Protein -1g   Calories -264

DAY 6

Celery Crunch Salad

Bok Choy Soup

Dried Chicken Breast a la "Carpaccio"

Stuffed Pork Tenderloin Wrapped in Bacon

Coconut Snowballs
Fat - 83g Carbs - 40g   Protein -126g Calories -1411

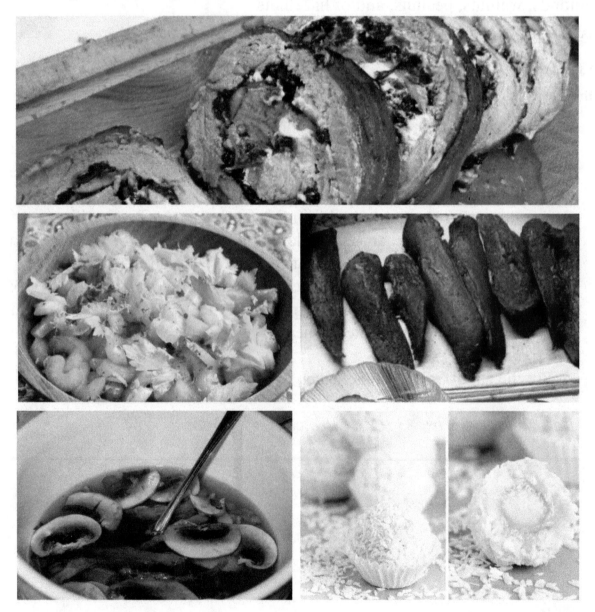

CELERY CRUNCH SALAD

4 serves | 10 min

Ingredients

8 stalks celery (with leaves)

1 green apple

¼ cup crumbled blue cheese

1 cup chopped pecans

¼ cup parsley

1 chopped green onion

¼ cup extra virgin olive oil

1 tablespoon Dijon mustard

½ lemon (juice)

2 tablespoons white wine vinegar

Directions

<u>Salad</u>

1. Wash and chop celery into medium slices. Place slices in a large bowl.
2. Wash and cut apple into thin slices. Add slices to the bowl.
3. Chop parsley and add to the bowl.
4. Chop pecans. Add the pecans to the bowl.
5. Add blue cheese, green onion to the mixture.
6. Drizzle the dressing over the top of the salad.

<u>Dressing</u>

1. In separate bowl, mix mustard, lemon juice, and vinegar.
2. Whisk the ingredients and drizzle with olive oil. Add salt and pepper.

Fat - 28g Carbs – 13g   Protein -5g   Calories -303

BOK CHOY SOUP
1 serves | 5 min

Ingredients

2 bok choy stalks

1 cup vegetable broth

1 teaspoon nutritional yeast

2 pinch garlic powder

2 pinch onion powder

salt and pepper to taste

Directions

1. Take a bowl. Mix all ingredients in it.
2. Place the bowl in a microwave for 3 minutes.

Fat - 2g   Carbs – 7g   Protein -9g   Calories -73

DRIED CHICKEN BREAST A LA "CARPACCIO"

4 serves | 6 h 10 min

Ingredients

2 1/3 pound chicken breast

5 teaspoons salt

2 teaspoons coriander

1/2 teaspoons spices, to taste

1 teaspoon black pepper

3 teaspoons sweet pepper

Paprika

Directions

1. Cut each half of a chilled breast lengthwise into two parts. You'll have 4 long thick pieces.
2. Pat each piece dry with a paper towel.
3. Mix the spices and crush before drying chicken.
4. Roll each chicken piece in spices until well coated and salt lightly.
5. Put the chicken in a container, pressing the pieces down.
6. Place the container in the refrigerator for 6-8 hours.
7. After cooling cut a small piece of rinse and taste. Taste a small piece of chicken to see if it is too salty. If it's not too salty, rinse the chicken under water. If it is salty, soak the chicken for 30 min. before rinsing. Then, rinse again and dry.
8. Cut the chicken into pieces, cover pieces in paprika. Then, string pieces on skewers for kebabs. Hang these skewers to dry at room temperature for 12-16 hours.

Fat - 7g   Carbs – 8g   Protein -54g   Calories -315

STUFFED PORK TENDERLOIN WRAPPED IN BACON

serves | 1 h

Ingredients

1 pound pork tenderloin

14 slices bacon

2 teaspoons minced garlic

½ small onion (2-4 ounces)

2 ounces spinach

3 ounces cream cheese

1 tablespoon olive oil

¾ teaspoon liquid smoke

¾ teaspoon dried thyme and rosemary

salt and pepper

For Vegetable Sauté

4 ounces chopped broccoli

½ orange bell pepper

½ cup diced tomatoes

½ teaspoon onion and garlic powder

salt and pepper

Directions

1. In a frying pan, cook onion in olive oil until soft (a few minutes).
2. Add garlic. Chop for 60 seconds. Then, add spinach, ¼ teaspoon dried thyme and rosemary and salt and pepper to taste.
3. Preheat oven to 355 °F.
4. Lay pork tenderloin on the cutting board. Pound it with meat hammer until flat. Shape tenderloin into a square and season with salt and pepper. Add liquid smoke.
5. Make a bacon weave the same size as the tenderloin.

6. Spread cream cheese and spinach on the pork tenderloin. Place these ingredients on top of bacon. Roll up.
7. Season stuffed pork with salt, pepper, ¼ teaspoon of thyme and rosemary.
8. Hold together the bacon ends with toothpicks if it's necessary. Place roll in the frying pan.
9. Bake it for 75-90 minutes.
10. For garnish stew broccoli, peppers, and tomatoes in the fat in the bottom of the pan after baking pork.

Fat - 43g Carbs – 4g   Protein -57g   Calories -655

COCONUT SNOWBALLS

5 serves | 10 min

Ingredients

2 ounces shredded coconut

1 ounce almond flour

1 ½ ounce agave syrup

Directions

1. Mix 1 ½ ounce shredded coconut, flour, and syrup in a food processor until well combined.
2. Make 10 balls using your hands.
3. Roll the balls in ½ ounce shredded coconut.

You can keep these balls in a sealed container in a fridge for one week.

Fat - 4g   Carbs – 8g   Protein -1g Calories -65

DAY 7

Avocado and Chicken Salad with Bacon
Cauliflower Cream Soup
Buffalo Chicken Meatballs
Beef Stew
Vegan Chocolate Turron
Fat - 136g   Carbs - 40g   Protein -127g Calories -1388

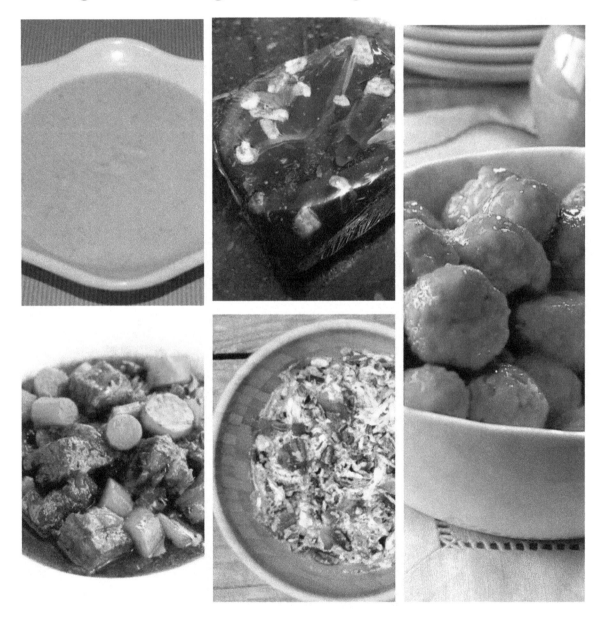

AVOCADO AND CHICKEN SALAD WITH BACON
4 serves | 15 min

Ingredients

1 slice bacon

½ medium avocado

¼ pound chicken breast

1 ounce Cheddar cheese

1 hard-boiled egg

½ pound Romaine lettuce

1 tablespoon olive oil

1 tablespoon apple cider vinegar

salt and pepper

Directions

1. Chop the lettuce. Place into salad bowl.
2. Chop bacon, avocado, chicken breast, Cheddar cheese, and egg. Place the ingredients atop the lettuce.
3. Add oil and vinegar. Sprinkle salt and pepper.

Fat - 13g   Carbs – 4g   Protein -9g Calories -189

CAULIFLOWER CREAM SOUP

2 serves | 35 min

Ingredients:

½ pound cauliflower

2 ounces onions

1 ounce butter

1 ounce cheese

1/3 pound chicken broth

1 ounce fatty cream

salt and pepper to taste

Directions:

1. Peel and cut onion well.
2. On the frying pan cook the onion until it is golden brown.
3. In a big pot, boil the cauliflower and, cook for 15 minutes.
4. Blend cooked cauliflower in the food processor.
5. Add chicken broth, fried onions, cream, chopped cauliflower in the saucepan. Add grated cheese. Boil for 10 minutes.
6. Add salt and spices to taste.

Fat - 19g   Carbs – 9g   Protein -9g   Calories -229

BUFFALO CHICKEN MEATBALLS

4 serves | 30 min

Ingredients

1 pound organic chicken

1 egg, beaten

2 green onions, chopped

1 celery stalk, chopped finely

1 tablespoon almond flour or coconut flour

1 tablespoon organic mayonnaise

1 teaspoon onion powder

1 teaspoon garlic powder

1 teaspoon natural salt

1 teaspoon pepper

1 cup buffalo sauce for wings

Directions

1. Preheat oven to 400 °F. Grease a baking sheet with coconut oil (or butter or avocado oil).
2. In a large bowl, mix all ingredients, except the buffalo sauce.
3. Make 2-inch balls from the mixture. Place the meatballs on the baking sheet. Bake for 15 min.
4. Remove the meatballs from the oven.
5. Place the meatballs in the skillet over the medium heat.
6. Add the buffalo sauce to the skillet. Cook until the sauce is warmed through.

Fat - 75g   Carbs – 8g   Protein -40g   Calories -333

BEEF STEW
6 serves | 4 h

Ingredients

5 pounds beef snack, tail

3 medium carrots

8 Campari tomatoes

2 medium onions

1 teaspoon tomato sauce

8 cloves garlic

2 teaspoons garlic powder

2 tablespoons apple cider vinegar

4 cups chicken broth

2 cups water

2 teaspoons onion powder

4 teaspoons salt

3 teaspoons crushed red pepper

2 teaspoons parsley

1 teaspoon cayenne

2 teaspoons black pepper

2 teaspoons basil

3 whole bay leaves, spices, to taste

Directions

1. Pell and cut carrots, tomatoes, onion, garlic into chunky pieces.
2. Preheat the frying pan over medium heat.
3.   Place vegetables and spices on the frying pan, stir and cook until translucent.
4. Replace the ingredients in the soup pot.
5.   Take another cast iron skillet. Place beef snack in it . Cook on both sides, until crispy.

6. Pour broth into the pot to the onion, carrot and garlic.
7. Add two cups of water, apple cider vinegar. Cook for 2-3 minutes. Stir.
8. Add tomatoes, tomato sauce. Stir well.
9. Submerge beef tails into the broth. Boil the ingredients.
10. Reduce the heat to a simmer. Cover the pot.
11. Slightly simmer on a low heat for 3 hours.
12. When meat is cooked, it will be very soft and tender.
13. Remove the bay leaves from the pot. Serve.

Fat - 22g Carbs – 9g   Protein -68g   Calories -531

VEGAN CHOCOLATE TURRON
8 serves | 15 min +chill time

Ingredients

1/3 pound dark chopped chocolate

1 tablespoon melted coconut oil

1 ounce unsalted raw hazelnuts

Directions

1. Place dark chocolate in a saucepan. Cook over medium heat, stirring occasionally until chocolate is melted.
2. Remove chocolate from the heat. Add hazelnuts, and combine well.
3. Pour the chocolate-hazelnuts mixture into lined rectangular dish.
4. Cool to room temperature. Chop the turron.
5. If it's too hot in the room, keep turron in the fridge.

Fat - 8g   Carbs – 10g   Protein -1g   Calories -106

WEEK 2

	Week 2				
MEAL	**Breakfast**	**Lunch**	**Snacks**	**Dinner**	**Dessert**
SUNDAY	Savory Bacon Cranberry Cheese Tartlets	Broccoli Cheese Soup	Avocado Chicken Roll	Roasted Turkey with Rosemary Thyme Gravy	"Ferrero Rocher" Keto Fat Bombs
MONDAY	Spinach and Artichoke Casserole	Keto Chicken Salad	Buffalo Deviled Eggs	Lamb Leg with Rosemary and Garlic	Keto Pizza
TUESDAY	Avocado and Chicken Salad with Bacon	Meat Soup	Chocolate Fat Bombs with Sunflower Seeds	Lamb Leg with Rosemary and Garlic	Light Coconut Chocolate Bombs
WEDNESDAY	Stuffed Mushrooms with Sausage	Chorizo Soup	Bacon and Cheese Cauliflower Muffins	Creole Shrimp	Georgian Pkhali
THURSDAY	Stuffed Pork Tenderloin Wrapped in Bacon	Chicken Curry Stew	Cheddar Crisps	Salmon and Asparagus with Onion-Mushroom Sauce	Pumpkin Cheesecake Mousse
FRIDAY	Walnuts Fennel and Goat Cheese Green Bean Salad	Mushrooms with Chicken and Spices	Buns with Oregano	Green Chile Pork Stew	Almond Cookies
SATURDAY	Shrimp and Greens Salad	French Onion Soup	Pesto Mushrooms	Beef Stew (low-carb)	Lemon and Blackberry Pudding

WEEK 2 SHOPPING LIST

PANTRY STAPLES	VEGETABLES
Butter	Avocados – 3 total
Almond flour - 1 lb	Artichoke hearts – 1 lb
Coconut flour – 1/3 cup	Brussels sprouts – 2 total
Coconut Milk – 2 pack	Green beans – 1 lb
	Onions – 13 total
DAIRY & MEAT	Lemon – 3 total
Heavy Cream – 10 oz	Cauliflower - 2 lb
Soft Cream Cheese – 4 containers (24 oz)	Carrots – 2 total
Goat cheese – 8 oz	Spinach – 11 oz
Cheddar Cheese – 20 oz	Broccoli – 32 oz frozen
Eggs – 23 total	Olives – 8 oz
Bacon slices – 54 oz	
Pork tenderloin – 1 lb	**OTHER**
Italian sausage – 8 oz	Hazelnuts – 12 oz
Chicken – 3 lb	Mushrooms – 30 oz
Chicken breast – 24 oz	Salmon - 1 lb
Gorgonzola cheese – oz	Shrimp – 1 lb
Mozzarella – 16 oz	Walnuts – 8 oz
Leg of bone – in lag – 8 lb	Champignons -12 oz
Turkey – 3 lb	
Ground pork - 2 lb	
Parmesan cheese grated – 9 oz	
Diced tomatoes – 3 lb	
Beef Stew – 1 lb	

DAY 8

Savory Bacon Cranberry Cheese Tartlets
Broccoli Cheese Soup
Avocado Chicken Roll
Roasted Turkey with Rosemary Thyme Gravy
"Ferrero Rocher" Keto Fat Bombs
Fat - 116g   Carbs -29g   Protein -152g Calories -1772

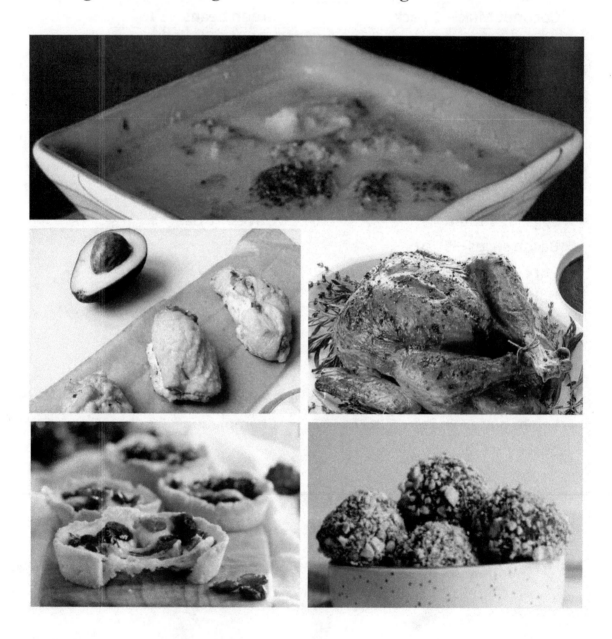

SAVORY BACON CRANBERRY CHEESE TARTLETS

6 serves | 30 min

Ingredients

Tart crust

1 cup blanched almond flour

1 egg

1/5 cup butter melted

sea salt

Filling

3 chopped bacon slices

½ cups cubed Mahon Menorca Semi-Cured Cheese

1/4 cup unsweetened dried cranberries

1 teaspoon fresh thyme leaves

salt

black pepper to taste

Directions

1. Preheat oven to 370 °F. Grease 6-cup muffin pan.
2. Combine the ingredients for the crust. Form dough.
3. Make 6 balls with your hands. Place one into each cup.
4. Press dough with a small glass to make the tart crusts.
5. Bake the crusts for 7 minutes until lightly golden. Remove them from the oven.
6. Fill the crusts with fried and chopped bacon, cubed Mahon Menorca cheese, and dried cranberries.
7. Sprinkle the tartlets with salt, pepper, and fresh thyme leaves.
8. Bake for 10 minutes or until cheese is completely melted.
9. Remove the tartlets and cool for 10 minutes.

Fat - 33g   Carbs – 7g   Protein -11g   Calories -360

BROCCOLI CHEESE SOUP

8 serves | 20 min

Ingredients

4 cups broccoli

4 cloves of minced garlic

3 ½ cups vegetable broth

1 cup heavy cream

3 cups shredded cheddar cheese

Directions

1. Saute garlic for 1 minute in a large pot over medium heat. Cook until fragrant.
2. Add chicken broth, chopped broccoli, heavy cream. Increase heat to a boil. After that reduce heat, simmer for 20 minutes until broccoli are tender.
3. Add shredded cheddar cheese gradually. Stir constantly until melted. Make very low heat to simmer. Remove the pot from the heat immediately once all the cheese is melted.

Fat - 20g Carbs – 5g   Protein -15g Calories -257

AVOCADO CHICKEN ROLL

1 serves | 15 min

Ingredients

¼ pound fried chicken breast

1 tablespoon mayonnaise

½ medium avocado

salt

pepper

Directions

1. Cut the chicken into thin long strips.
2. Cut avocado into medium slices, put them in a plate, mix with mayonnaise and salt and pepper to taste.
3. Put avocado mixture on the meat strips. Roll strips.

Fat - 30g Carbs – 13g   Protein -36g   Calories -449

ROASTED TURKEY WITH ROSEMARY THYME GRAVY

6 serves | 4 h 30 min

Ingredients

Roasted Turkey

4 pounds whole turkey

½ small onion

1 small lemon

1/8 cup minced garlic

1 teaspoon dried rosemary

2 chopped stalks green onions

Turkey Coating

2 tablespoons melted butter

1/2 teaspoons cayenne

1 teaspoon chicken herb seasoning

Gravy

Leftover parts of turkey

1/6 cup chicken stock

1 ½ cups water

1 teaspoon Worcestershire

1 stalks green onions

2 Brussels sprouts

1 tablespoon bacon fat

2 sprigs fresh thyme

1 bay leaf

1/8 teaspoon xanthan gum

1/8 cup heavy cream

Salt and pepper

Directions

1.   Preheat oven to 325 ºF. Stuff the turkey with onion, lemon, minced garlic, dried rosemary, and chopped green onions.
2.   Mix the coating ingredients. Brush the turkey with this mixture.
3.   Bake turkey for 150 minutes.
4.   Boil the turkey innards in water and chicken broth for 1 hour.
5.   Add brussels sprouts. Green onion, Worcestershire, salt, and pepper to the gravy. Boil for 30-45 minutes. Then blend gravy.
6.   Add sprigs of fresh thyme, bay leaf, and heavy cream. Bring to a rolling boil.
7.   Stir Continuously. Let gravy reduce for 15-20 minutes. It should be relatively thick. Add the xanthan gum, and mix well.
8.   Let turkey rest. Serve with gravy.

Fat - 20g Carbs – 3g   Protein -88g Calories -566

"FERRERO ROCHER" KETO FAT BOMBS

7 serves | 1 h 15 min

Ingredients

1 1/2 ounce ground hazelnuts

1 ounce coconut oil

Erythritol powder

1 ½ ounce sugar-free chocolate

1/2 teaspoons sugar-free vanilla extract

1 teaspoon cocoa powder

Chopped hazelnuts and 7 whole hazelnuts

Directions

1. Melt the sugar-free chocolate in a double boiler.
2. Melt the coconut oil in the microwave if needed.
3. Add the chopped hazelnuts, powdered erythritol, melted coconut oil, cocoa powder, and vanilla extract into a food processor and blend on high for approximately 30–45 seconds.
4. Add the melted chocolate and blend for another 15 seconds.
5. Cool down the mixture in the freezer, then form 7 small balls with your hands.
6. Push a whole hazelnut into the middle of each fat bomb and roll the balls in chopped hazelnuts. Refrigerate.

Fat - 14g Carbs – 1g   Protein -2g   Calories -140

DAY 9

Spinach and Artichoke Casserole
Keto Chicken Salad
Buffalo Deviled Eggs
Lamb Leg with Rosemary and Garlic
Keto Pizza
Fat - 138g   Carbs -27g   Protein -151g Calories -1972

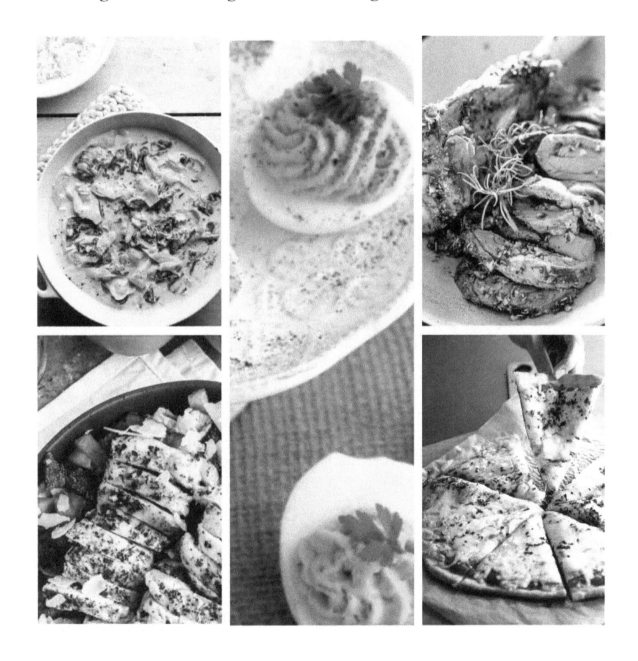

SPINACH AND ARTICHOKE CASSEROLE

8 serves | 50 min

Ingredients

½ pound cream cheese

¼ cup homemade mayonnaise

1/3 pound shredded Parmesan cheese

1 tablespoon minced garlic

1 teaspoon crushed basil

1 pound artichoke hearts

½ pound spinach

½ pound Mozzarella cheese

Salt and paper to taste

Directions

1. Preheat oven to 350 ºF
2. Melt cream cheese in the microwave.
3. Add the mayo to the melted cream cheese. Combine the ingredients.
4. Add shredded Parmesan, garlic, and basil. Mix the ingredients. Add salt and pepper.
5. Chop the artichoke and add it to the other ingredients. Mix well.
6. Cut the spinach and combine with the artichoke mixture.
7. Grease a baking sheet with oil. Placed the mixture on baking sheet.
8. Cover the top of the dish with shredded mozzarella.

Bake the casserole for 30 minutes.

Fat - 17g Carbs – 10g   Protein -12g   Calories -233

KETO CHICKEN SALAD
1 serves | 20 min

Ingredients

2/3 pound chicken breast

3 ounces thin-cut bacon slices

½ pound avocado

½ ounce mixed leaf greens

2 tablespoons Paleo Ranch Dressing

Duck fat for greasing

Directions

1. Preheat the oven to 400 ºF.
2. Crisp the chicken breasts. Season with salt and pepper.
3. Grease pan with fat. Place breasts skin side down on the pan. Fry for 5-6 minutes. Flip the chicken and cook 30 seconds. Than transfer pan in the oven. Cook 10-15 minutes, until chicken is cooked through.
4. Place the slices bacon on the bake sheet. Bake the bacon slices in the oven until crispy. Alternatively, crisp the bacon in a frying pan.
5. Remove chicken from the oven. Cool for 5 minutes.
6. Slice the avocado and cooked chicken.
7. Place leafy greens on the plate. Add avocado, crispy bacon and sliced chicken.
8. Top with Ranch dressing.

Fat - 48g   Carbs – 12g Protein -48g   Calories -627

BUFFALO DEVILED EGGS

6 serves | 20 min

Ingredients

6 hard boiled chicken eggs, large

1/3 pound boiled and chopped chicken

¼ onion

¼ cup blue cheese crumbles

¼ cup Franks Buffalo Wing Sauce

1 small chopped celery

2 tablespoons blue cheese dressing

Directions

1. Boil the eggs.
2. Chop the chicken and celery.
3. Peel cooked and cooled eggs. Cut them in half lengthwise. Separate the yolks from the egg whites and place yolks in mixing bowl.
4. Add chicken, celery, blue cheese, Franks Buffalo Wing Sauce and dressing to yolks.
5. Press the onion and add juice to the bowl. Mix all the ingredients.
6. Stuff the egg whites with yolk mixture using a fork or spoon. You can also pipe the yolks into the whites using a Ziploc bag with the tip cut off.

Fat - 12g Carbs – 2g   Protein -29g   Calories -152

LAMB LEG WITH ROSEMARY AND GARLIC
6 serves | 2 h 30 min

Ingredients

4 pounds leg of bone-in lamb

1 sliced cloves garlic

1 thinly sliced lemons

3 fresh rosemary sprigs

salt and pepper

1 teaspoon oil

Directions

1. Preheat the oven to 350 ºF. Grease the baking sheet.
2. With a knife, make 1/2-inch-deep slits all over the lamb (about 25 cuts).
3. Stuff the garlic into the slits.
4. Mix 1 teaspoon salt and ½ teaspoon pepper. Season lamb with this mixture. Leave meat at room temperature for 45 minutes.
5. Place the slices lemon on the sheet so they overlap. They will keep the meat from burning. Place one rosemary sprigs on the lemon and lamb. Place 2 sprigs on the top of the lamb.
6. Bake lamb for 1 ½ to 2 hours. Baste with the pan juice every 15 minutes.
7. Loosely tent the lamb with the foil. Let rest. Slice perpendicular to the bone

Fat - 56g Carbs – 2g   *Protein -58g   Calories -800*

KETO PIZZA
8 serves | 1 h

Ingredients

Sauce

1/3 cup canned sugar-free crushed tomatoes

1 teaspoon olive oil

1 small clove garlic, minced

A pinch of kosher salt

Keto Dough

1 ½ cups shredded Mozzarella

2 tablespoons full-fat sour cream

2/3 cup almond flour

2 large eggs, lightly beaten

A pinch of kosher salt

Olive oil

Toppings

1/3 cup shredded whole-milk Mozzarella

Crushed red pepper flakes and dried oregano, for sprinkling

Directions

Sauce

1. Combine the tomatoes, minced garlic, and salt in a small bowl.
2. Let the mixture sit for 30 min. at room temperature.

Dough

1. Place the cheese and sour cream in a large microwave-safe bowl.
2. Microwave the ingredients in one-minute intervals, stirring until the cheese is melted. Cool the mixture slightly.

3. Add the eggs, flour, and ¼ teaspoon of salt to the cheese mixture. Mix with your hands until a stretchy, slightly wet dough forms.

Pizza

1. Adjust an oven rack to the low position and place a baking sheet on it.
2. Preheat oven to 450 ˚F.
3. Grease a piece of parchment paper with olive oil.
4. Lightly coat your hands in oil and place the dough on the parchment, patting into a ¼-inch-thick rectangle. Make the edges a bit thicker to create a crust all around.
5. Place the dough on the baking sheet. Bake until puffy and golden. Cook about 15 min.
6. Remove the dough from the oven and top with sauce and mozzarella. Bake pizza until it's heated through and cheese is melted, about 5 min.
7. Remove the dough from the oven.
8. Sprinkle with pepper flakes, salt, and oregano.

Fat - 5g   Carbs – 1g   Protein -4g   Calories -160

DAY 10

Avocado and Chicken Salad with Bacon

Meat Soup

Chocolate Fat Bombs with Sunflower Seeds

Lamb Leg with Rosemary and Garlic

Light Coconut Chocolate Bombs

Fat - 279 Carbs -25, Protein – 97, Calories - 2166

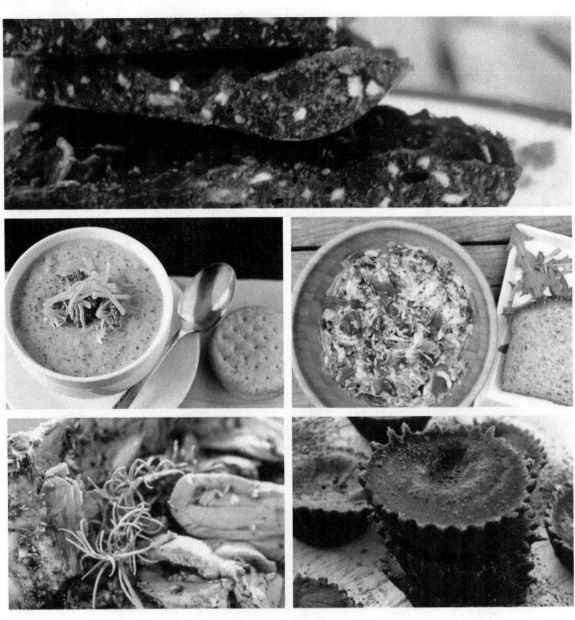

AVOCADO AND CHICKEN SALAD WITH BACON

4 serves | 20 min

Ingredients

1 slice bacon

½ medium avocado

¼ pound chicken breast

1 ounce Cheddar cheese

1 hard-boiled egg

½ pound Romaine lettuce

1 tablespoon olive oil

1 tablespoon apple cider vinegar

salt and pepper

Directions

1. Chop the lettuce. Place into salad bowl.
2. Chop bacon, avocado, chicken breast, Cheddar cheese, and egg. Place the ingredients atop the lettuce.
3. Add oil and vinegar. Sprinkle salt and pepper.

Fat - 13g Carbs – 4g   Protein -9g   Calories -189

MEAT SOUP
6 serves | 50 min

Ingredients

8 slices bacon

4 cups fried broccoli

½ large sliced onion

2 cups shredded cheddar cheese

2 cups chicken broth

¼ cup shredded Parmesan

2 tablespoons butter

2 tablespoons coconut flour

½ cup heavy cream

2 teaspoons minced garlic

½ teaspoon salt

1 teaspoon cayenne pepper

Directions

1. Fry bacon over medium heat for 5-7 minutes in a frying pan.
2. Chop the onion.
3. Remove the bacon on a paper towel. Leave 3 tablespoons of bacon fat in the pan.
4. Add butter, onion, and garlic to the pan, and fry for 4-5 minutes until onion is translucent.
5. Add coconut flour to the pan and cook for 1 minute.
6. Mix cream and milk in a bowl. Add the mixture to the pan and wait until it starts to bubble. Mix well and reduce heat to medium level.
7. Add cheddar cheese and parmesan to the pan, and mix well. Cook for 2-3 minutes on low heat, then add broccoli and cook for 2-3 minutes.
8. Add bacon and cook for 5 minutes. Turn off the heat.
9. Mix the ingredients in the pan with the blender, then add broth, cayenne pepper and mix again.

10. Turn on medium heat. Simmer the soup for 20-30 minutes, stirring it every 5 minutes.

Fat - 40g   Carbs – 8g   Protein -20g   Calories -476

CHOCOLATE FAT BOMBS WITH SUNFLOWER SEEDS

4 serves | 40 min

Ingredients

3 ½ ounces of sunflower seeds, roasted and ground

7 ounces butter, melted

2 teaspoons sweetener (for example, Stevie)

3 tablespoons cocoa powder

vanilla or vanilla extract to taste

Directions

1. Mix all dry ingredients.
2. Add melted butter and vanilla, and stir well.
3. Pour the mixture into silicone molds and refrigerate.

Note: It's essentially a bombshell. There are 91.7% fat, 4% protein, 4.2% carbohydrate.

Fat - 24g Carbs – 3g   *Protein -3g*   *Calories -232*

LAMB LEG WITH ROSEMARY AND GARLIC

6 serves | 2 h 30 min

Ingredients

4 pounds leg of bone-in lamb

1 sliced cloves garlic

1 thinly sliced lemons

3 fresh rosemary sprigs

salt and pepper

1 teaspoon oil

Cooking

1. Preheat the oven to 350°F. Grease the baking sheet.
2. With a knife, make 1/2-inch-deep slits all over the lamb (about 25 cuts).
3. Stuff the garlic into the slits.
4. Mix 1 teaspoon salt and ½ teaspoon pepper. Season lamb with this mixture. Leave meat at room temperature for 45 minutes.
5. Place the slices lemon on the sheet so they overlap. They will keep the meat from burning. Place one rosemary sprigs on the lemon and lamb. Place 2 sprigs on the top of the lamb.
6. Bake lamb for 1 ½ to 2 hours. Baste with the pan juice every 15 minutes.
7. Loosely tent the lamb with the foil. Let rest. Slice perpendicular to the bone

Fat - 56g Carbs – 2g   *Protein -58g   Calories -800*

LIGHT COCONUT CHOCOLATE BOMBS

10 serves | 10 min

Ingredients

1 cups of macadamia nuts, salted

1–2 tablespoons coconut oil (melted, for most solid fat bombs)

1/2 teaspoons vanilla extract (optional)

3 teaspoons powdered sweetener

1 ounce cocoa powder

Directions

1. Put the macadamia nuts in a food processor or high-power blender and pulse them into small pieces.
2. Add melted coconut oil and vanilla, if using, to the nuts. Mash until a butter is formed.
3. Pour the cocoa powder and sweetener onto the paste gradually while stirring. Mix the ingredients until smooth.
4. Place pieces of parchment paper into mini-cupcake molds. Spoon the dough evenly into the molds.
5. Freeze for about 30 minutes to harden.

Note: use salted macadamia nuts. If you have unsalted, add sea salt to taste.

Fat - 45g Carbs – 9g   Protein -8g   Calories -469

DAY 11

Low calories day. Try to limit physical activity today.

Stuffed Mushrooms with Sausage
Chorizo Soup
Bacon and Cheese Cauliflower Muffins
Creole Shrimp
Georgian Pkhali
Fat -123 g   Carbs -34 g   Protein -63g   Calories -1138

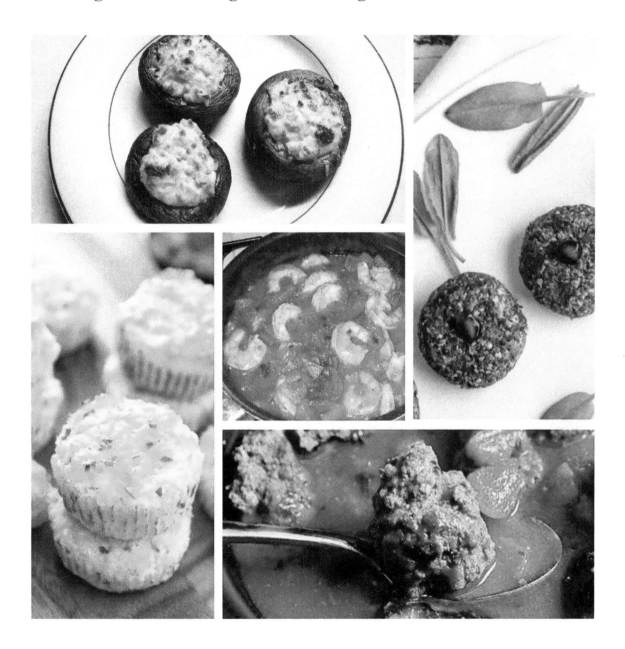

STUFFED MUSHROOMS WITH SAUSAGE
6 serves | 45 min

Ingredients

10-12 large mushrooms

½ pound Italian sausage, sliced

1 small onion

1/3 pound grated Parmesan cheese

1/8 cup Italian bread crumbs

1/2 teaspoons minced garlic

1/2 teaspoons chopped fresh parsley

Directions

1. Preheat oven to 350 ºF.
2. Hollow out mushroom caps, save scrapings.
3. Heat frying pan over medium-high heat. Add sausage, onion, and reserved mushroom scrapings. Cook and stir the ingredients 4-6 minutes until sausage is browned.
4. Drain and discard liquid. And fry again.
5. Add 4 ounces Parmesan cheese, bread crumbs, garlic, and parsley to sausage mixture. Cook 3-5 minutes.
6. Cool sausage mixture. Stuff each mushroom cap with mixture. Place the stuffed caps on a baking sheet. Bake for 12 minutes. Then sprinkle remaining 2 ounces Parmesan cheese over mushrooms. Bake until cheese is melted and bubbling, about 3 minutes.

Fat - 10g Carbs – 3g   *Protein -11g   Calories -142*

CHORIZO SOUP

6 serves | 1 h 10 min

Ingredients

1 teaspoon extra virgin olive oil

2 onions, finely chopped

2 cloves of garlic, minced

1 green bell pepper, finely chopped

3 ounces chorizo

3 cups jarred or fresh tomatoes, finely diced

2 cups chicken broth

½ red pepper flakes

1 teaspoon fresh cilantro to taste

¾ cup Cheddar cheese to taste

organic tortilla to taste

Directions

1. Chop onions, garlic, tomatoes, and pepper with a knife. Or use a food processor until finely chopped.
2. Take a stock pot, place it over medium-high heat.
3. Cut and crumble the chorizo.
4. Place garlic, bell pepper, chorizo, onions in the pot.
5. Saute soup's ingredients until onion is brown.
6. Stir tomatoes, broth, pepper flakes in the stock pot.

Fat - 12g   *Carbs – 10g*   *Protein -10g*   *Calories -202*

BACON AND CHEESE CAULIFLOWER MUFFINS

6 serves | 45 min

Ingredients

1/3 pound chopped cauliflower

2 ounces grated Cheddar cheese

1 large chicken eggs

4 pieces bacon

½ ounce almond flour

½ ounce feta cheese

1/4 teaspoon baking powder

1 teaspoon garlic powder

1 teaspoon celery

1 teaspoon oregano

1 teaspoon paprika

Salt and pepper, to taste

Directions

1. Preheat oven to 400 °F.
2. Grind the cauliflower and place in a large bowl. Add the dry ingredients, bacon, and cheese.
3. Add eggs, mix thoroughly until mixture forms.
4. Place the mixture in cupcake molds.
5. Sprinkle with feta cheese.
6. Bake for 35 min.

Fat - 8g   Carbs – 3g   Protein -8g   Calories -115

CREOLE SHRIMP

4 serves | 30 min

Ingredients

½ pound large shrimp

½ pound smoked sausage, (can be replaced with shrimp)

1/4 cup olive or canola oil

1/4 cup celery, diced

1 medium onion, chopped

1 small bell pepper, chopped

2 teaspoons garlic, minced

1 bay leaf

1-2 teaspoons fresh thyme

2 teaspoons creole seasoning or more

½ -1 pound stew tomatoes or 2-3 fresh tomatoes

2 cups or more broth/water

1 teaspoon Worcestershire sauce

1 teaspoon bouillon powder, optional

1-2 green onions, chopped

2 tablespoons parsley, chopped

Directions

1.   Sauté shrimp with creole seasoning and 1 tablespoon oil over medium heat in a heavy bottomed dutch for about 1- 2 minutes.
2.   Add sausage and saute until browned on both sides. Remove aside.
3.   Fry onions, celery, green pepper, thyme and garlic with remaining oil, while stiring for about 2-3 minutes.
4.   Top up leaf creole spice, tomatoes, chicken broth, and Worcestershire sauce. Simmer for 10-15 minutes. Add bouillon as needed.
5.   Pout out shrimp with sausage to the dutch, mix all ingredients and cook for about 2-3 minutes.
6.   Serve with white rice or fettuccine garnishing parsley.

Fat - 68g Carbs – 9g   Protein -21g   Calories -391

GEORGIAN PKHALI

3 serves | 2 h 15 min

Ingredients

1 cup walnuts

1 bunch spinach, roughly chopped

1 bunch parsley, roughly chopped

2 cloves garlic, peeled

½ teaspoon salt

Lemon juice to taste

Directions

1. Soak the nuts in water for at least 2 hours.
2. Drain and rinse the nuts, then blend in a food processor.
3. Peel the garlic.
4. Cut the greens.
5. Add garlic and greens. Blend until a homogeneous mixture forms.
6. Add lemon juice and salt to taste.
7. Roll into medium balls.

Fat - 25g   Carbs – 9g   Protein -14g   Calories -288

DAY 12

Stuffed Pork Tenderloin Wrapped in Bacon
Chicken Curry Stew
Cheddar Crisps
Salmon and Asparagus with Onion-Mushroom Sauce
Pumpkin Cheesecake Mousse
Fat -162 g   Carbs - 25g   Protein -121g Calories -2072

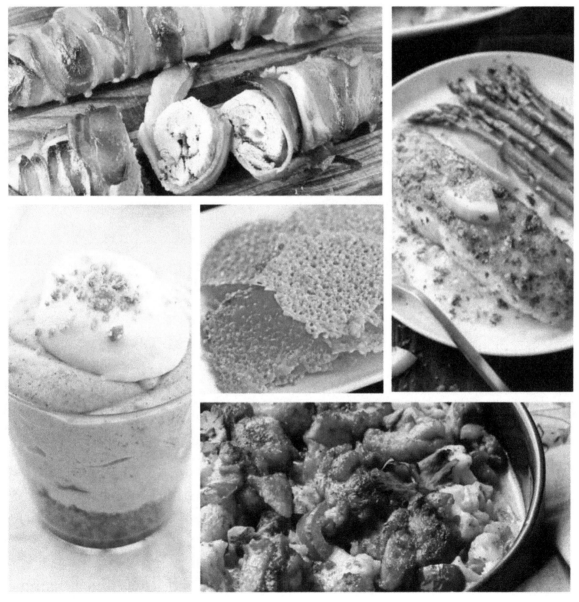

STUFFED PORK TENDERLOIN WRAPPED IN BACON

4 serves | 1 h

Ingredients

1 pound pork tenderloin

14 slices bacon

2 teaspoons minced garlic

½ small onion

2 ounces spinach

3 ounces cream cheese

1 tablespoon olive oil

¾ teaspoon liquid smoke

¾ teaspoon dried thyme and rosemary

salt and pepper

For Vegetable Sauté

1/3 pound chopped broccoli

½ orange bell pepper

½ cup decide tomatoes

½ teaspoon onion and garlic powder

salt and pepper

Directions

1. In a frying pan, cook onion in olive oil until soft (a few minutes).
2. Add garlic. Chop for 60 seconds. Then, add spinach, ¼ teaspoon dried thyme and rosemary and salt and pepper to taste.
3. Preheat oven to 355 ºF.
4. Lay pork tenderloin on the cutting board. Pound it with meat hammer until flat. Shape tenderloin into a square and season with salt and pepper. Add liquid smoke.
5. Make a bacon weave the same size as the tenderloin.

6. Spread cream cheese and spinach on the pork tenderloin. Place these ingredients on top of bacon. Roll up.
7. Season stuffed pork with salt, pepper, ¼ teaspoon of thyme and rosemary.
8. Hold together the bacon ends with toothpicks if it's necessary. Place roll in the frying pan.
9. Bake it for 75-90 minutes.
10. For garnish stew broccoli, peppers, and tomatoes in the fat in the bottom of the pan after baking pork.

Fat - 43g   Carbs – 4g   Protein -57g   Calories -655

CHICKEN CURRY STEW

serves | 40 min

Ingredients

1 ½ pound boneless chicken thighs

2 tablespoons curry powder

2 teaspoons garlic powder

1/3 cup coconut oil

1 pound cauliflower

1 green bell pepper

1 and ½ cups coconut milk

salt and pepper

¼ cup fresh cilantro/parsley

Directions

1. Cut chicken thighs into medium pieces.
2. Cut cauliflower, peppers into small pieces.
3. Heat coconut oil in the big frying pan or a wok.
4. Add curry and garlic powder. Fry for 1-2 minutes.
5. Add chicken to the skillet, add salt and pepper.
6. Sauté the ingredients for 5 minutes, while stirring often. Cook until golden brown and cooked through.
7. Remove from the pan, keep chicken warm.
8. Place cauliflower, bell pepper in the skillet. Fry vegetables on medium high heat for 3-5 minutes.
9. Add coconut milk to the vegetables, cook for 5-10 minutes.
10. Add salt, pepper, fried chicken to the pan and cook for 1 minute.
11. Use chopped cilantro for serving.

Fat - 68g   Carbs – 9g   Protein -33g   Calories -781

CHEDDAR CRISPS

4 serves | 15 min

Ingredients

4 tablespoons shredded Cheddar cheese

Directions

1. Preheat oven to 350 ºF.
2. Line bake sheet with parchment paper.
3. Drop the shredded cheese on paper. Make sure that there are 2 inches between the drops of the cheese.
4. Bake 10-15 minutes until the edges of the crisps brown.
5. Turn off the oven, remove the sheet. Cool the crisps for 10-15 minutes.

Fat - 2g   Carbs – 0g   Protein -2g   Calories -28

SALMON AND ASPARAGUS WITH ONION-MUSHROOM SAUCE

4 serves | 40 min

Ingredients

1 pound salmon

¼ pound champignons

1 onion

1 garlic clove

2 tablespoons olive oil

½ cup sesame oil

salt

basil

pepper

Directions

Marinade

Mix sesame oil with finely chopped garlic, basil, pepper, and salt.

Salmon and Asparagus

1. Cut the salmon, and put into a small saucepan. Pour the marinade over fish and chill in the refrigerator for an hour.
2. Preheat the oven to 355 ºF. Cover a baking sheet with foil.
3. Put the slices of salmon and washed asparagus on the baking sheet. Cover them with foil.
4. Bake fish and vegetables in the oven for 15-20 minutes.
5. Wash, peel, and cut champignons. Mince the onion. Fry the ingredients in olive oil until browned.
6. Remove the fish and asparagus from the oven, and top with mushroom and onion mixture. Bake for another 10 minutes.

Fat - 42g   Carbs – 3g   Protein -25g   Calories -478

PUMPKIN CHEESECAKE MOUSSE

6 serves | 10 min + chill time

Ingredients

1/3 pound softened cream cheese

½ pound unsweetened pumpkin puree

1/3 cup erythritol

1 teaspoon pure vanilla extract

1 tablespoon pumpkin pie spice

1/2 cup heavy cream

Directions

1. In a large mixing bowl, combine the cream cheese and pumpkin puree by hand. The mixture must be creamy, smooth, and without clumps.
2. Add vanilla, spices, erythritol, and heavy cream to the pumpkin mixture. Combine well.
3. The mousse must set in the refrigerator before it can be served.

Fat - 8g Carbs – 9g   Protein -4g   Calories -130

DAY 13

Walnuts Fennel and Goat Cheese Green Bean Salad
Mushrooms with Chicken and Spices
Buns with Oregano
Green Chile Pork Stew
Almond Cookies
Fat - 73g Carbs - 35g   Protein -75g   Calories -1210

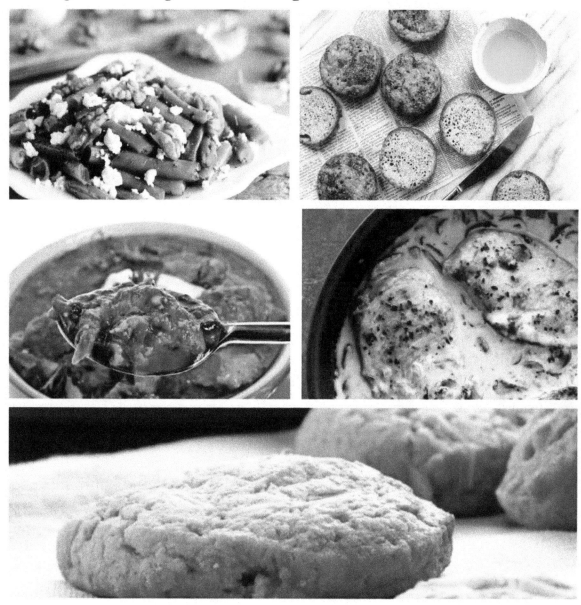

WALNUTS FENNEL AND GOAT CHEESE GREEN BEAN SALAD

6 serves | 40 min

Ingredients

1 tablespoon Dijon mustard

1 tablespoon white wine vinegar

1/2 teaspoons kosher salt

¼ teaspoon freshly ground black pepper

1/5 cup extra-virgin olive oil

1 pound trimmed green beans

1 small fennel bulb

1/2 cup walnuts

½ pound fresh Goat cheese

Directions

<u>Salad</u>

1. Boil salted water in a large saucepan. Add the green beans. Cook for 6-8 minutes.
2. Drain and cool under cold water.
3. Slice the fennel bulb into half-moons.
4. Toast and coarsely chop walnuts.
5. Crumble the goat cheese.
6. Combine the green beans, fennel, and walnuts. Before serving add the goat cheese.
7. Top with dressing.

<u>Dressing</u>

Whisk mustard, salt, vinegar, and pepper. Add the oil and combine.

Fat – 27g Carbs – 11g Protein -17g   *Calories -228*

MUSHROOMS WITH CHICKEN AND SPICES

4 serves | 2 h

Ingredients

2/3 pound ceps

½ pound raw chicken meat

1 cup chicken broth

1 tablespoon butter

2 tablespoons fatty whipped cream

1 clove of garlic

thyme

basil

oregano

salt

pepper

Directions

1. Wash and peel ceps well. Separate the caps from the legs.
2. Preheat the frying pan. Add mushrooms and fry for 5 minutes over low heat.
3. Cut chicken into large chunks. Add them to the mushrooms.
4. Add the broth. Season the ingredients with finely chopped garlic, a pinch of basil, thyme, oregano, pepper and salt.
5. Simmer for about 1.5 hours on low heat. Then, add butter and whipped cream.

Fat – 7g   Carbs – 7g   Protein -19g   Calories -173

BUNS WITH OREGANO

6 serves | 30 min

Ingredients

4 eggs

4 tablespoons olive oil

2 ounces almond flour

¼ teaspoon salt

1 tablespoon dried oregano

Directions

1. Preheat oven to 390 ºF.
2. Thoroughly mix the eggs, olive oil, flour, ¾ of the oregano, and the salt.
3. Pour the mixture into a 6-cup muffin mold.
4. Sprinkle with the remaining oregano.
5. Bake for 25 min. Then, cool at room temperature before removing the buns from molds.

Fat – 11g   Carbs – 1g   Protein -7g   Calories -131

GREEN CHILE PORK STEW
8 serves | 1 h 45 min

Ingredients

2 pounds pork loin

2 teaspoons ground cumin

2 teaspoons granulated garlic

1 teaspoon pure ground chile powder (to taste)

2 ounces chopped onion

2 cloves garlic

1 ½ pound can whole hatch green chilies and liquid

3 tablespoons oil

2 cups water

poached eggs optional

salt to taste

Directions

1. Cut pork loin into cubes.
2. Preheat oil in a big frying pan. Fry pork until brown.
3. Add spices to the pork. Cook until fragrant.
4. At the same time chop garlic and onion. Place ingredients in a food processor.
5. Add canned chilies to the food processor. Mix and make thick chunky paste.
6. Add chili and onion mixture to the pork. Pour the liquid of canned chilies.
7. Pour two cups of water.
8. Stir the ingredients and make low-heat. Cover the pan with a lid.
9. Simmer the stew for 60-90 minutes until pork is tender.
10. Add a little water during the last hour cooking.
11. Before finishing, add salt to taste.
12. Serve stew with the poached eggs.

Fat – 10g   Carbs – 4g   Protein -20g   Calories -182

ALMOND COOKIES

4 serves | 45 min

Ingredients

2 cups almond flour

1/2 cup erythritol

1/4 cup butter

2 chicken eggs

1 teaspoon extract of vanilla

1 teaspoon cinnamon

Salt and halves of almonds

Directions

1. Preheat the oven to 355 ºF.
2. While the oven is heating, mix almond flour, erythritol, cinnamon, and a pinch of salt in a bowl.
3. Beat the eggs in a small bowl. Add butter and vanilla. Stir.
4. Mix the dry ingredients with the egg mixture until evenly combined.
5. Form dough into small circles using a spoon.
6. Decorate circles with half an almond.
7. Line a baking sheet with parchment paper coated in butter. Put the cookies on it.

Bake for 10-15 minutes.

Fat – 18g   Carbs – 12g   Protein -12g   Calories -496

DAY 14

Shrimp and Greens Salad
French Onion Soup
Pesto Mushrooms
Beef Stew (low-carb)
Lemon and Blackberry Pudding
Fat - 121g   Carbs - 24g   Protein -63g   Calories -1414

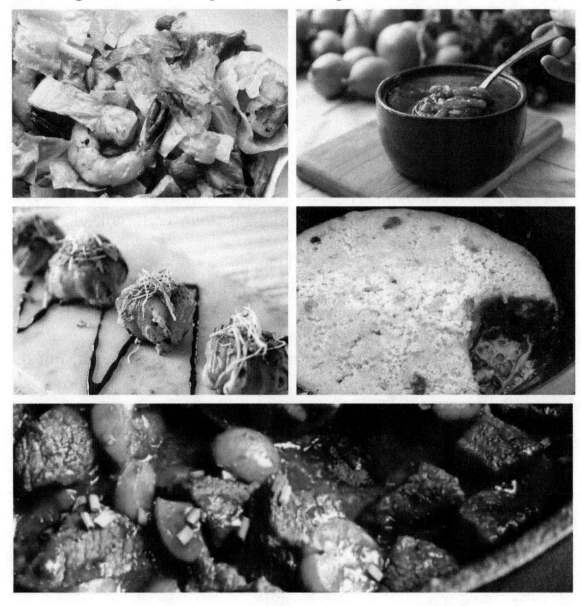

SHRIMP AND GREENS SALAD
4 serves | 20 min

Ingredients

½ pound peeled frozen shrimp

2 ounces salad

1 ounce olives

2 tablespoons butter

2 tablespoons olive oil

1 garlic clove

lemon juice

salt

pepper

Directions

1. Thaw the shrimp at room temperature or rinse with hot water. If you chose the second method, then use a colander. Rinse shrimp carefully.
2. Transfer the shrimps to a deep plate, add finely chopped garlic, lemon juice, salt and pepper. Mix well. Marinate the shrimp for 5-10 minutes.
3. Pre-heat a pan and add butter. Squeeze the shrimp a little. Lay shrimp in the frying pan. Fry the shrimp for 8-10 minutes.
4. Cool the shrimp.
5. Roughly chop the lettuce leaves. Put chopped leaves onto a large plate.
6. Add the shrimp and olives.
7. Season the ingredients with olive oil. Add salt and pepper to taste.

Fat – 14g   Carbs – 1g   Protein -9g   Calories -158

FRENCH ONION SOUP

8 serves | 1 h

Ingredients

¾ cup expeller-pressed coconut oil (or butter)

3-4 large sweet onions, sliced

6-10 minced cloves of fresh garlic

2 tablespoons arrowroot powder

½ cup red wine

2-3 teaspoons dried thyme

5 large bay leaves

1 ¼ teaspoon sea salt

½ teaspoon black pepper

½ teaspoon garlic powder

½ teaspoon onion powder

½ teaspoon garlic powder

½ t teaspoon onion powder

7 cups organic beef stock

Directions

1.   In a large saucepan place the coconut oil. Add thinly sliced onion, garlic. Cover the saucepan and stir occasionally. Cook for about 10 minutes over medium heat until onions are translucent.
2.   Add arrowroot powder for coating the onions.
3.   Add red wine, stirring around. Cook for 3-4 minutes to burn off the alcohol.
4.   Add spices and stir.
5.   Add beef stock and cook for 5-7 minutes.
6.   Reduce the heat to medium-low, simmer for 45 minutes.
7.   Remove from heat. Serve.
8.   Top the soup with cheese (Parmesan or Swiss) to taste.

Fat – 14g   Carbs – 1g   Protein -9g   Calories -158

PESTO MUSHROOMS

5 serves | 45 min

Ingredients

½ pound champignon

2/3 pound bacon

3 ounces cream cheese, softened

1 ounce pesto with basil

Directions

1. Preheat oven to 350 °F.
2. In a bowl, mix the cream cheese with the pesto sauce.
3. Place the bacon strips on a cutting board and cut strips in half lengthwise.
4. Peel the mushrooms and remove the stems.
5. Fill each mushroom cap with the cream cheese mixture and pesto.
6. Wrap a narrow strip of bacon around each mushroom. Wind the second strip around each cap in the other direction, so the mushroom is covered with bacon.
7. Place the mushrooms on the baking sheet and put in preheated oven.
8. Bake for 20-30 min. until the bacon is crispy and a pleasant golden brown.

Fat – 33g   Carbs – 3g   Protein -25g   Calories -409

BEEF STEW (LOW-CARB)

4 serves | 1 h 10 min

Ingredients

1 pound beef short rib

4 cloves garlic

2 cups beef broth

¼ pound carrot

1/4 teaspoon pink himalayan salt

¼ pound onion

¼ pound radishes

1/2 teaspoons xanthan gum

1/4 teaspoon pepper

1 tablespoon butter

1 tablespoon coconut oil

Directions

1.   Put chopped ribs along with salt and pepper on the heated large saucepan with coconut oil and brown them from all sides. Once cooked, set aside.
2.   Boil chopped onions along with garlic and butter. Mix it with broth when onions are tender.
3.   Add xanthan gum and combine.
4.   Put meat in the boiling broth and cook for 30 minutes with the lid closed.
5.   After that time, add chopped carrots and radishes and boil for another 30 minutes. Stir it during that time.
6.   Once the broth has thickened, the dish is ready. You can add water or bullion, if it is very thick.
7.   Stew should be served warm.

Fat – 37g   Carbs – 6g   Protein -19g   Calories -432

LEMON AND BLACKBERRY PUDDING

6 serves | 1 h 10 min

Ingredients

2 ounces coconut flour

5 chicken eggs

2 tablespoons butter

2 tablespoons coconut oil

2 tablespoons oily cream

2 tablespoons erythritol

1 lemon

2 teaspoons lemon juice

1/2 cup blackberries

1/4 teaspoon baking powder

10 drops liquid stevia

Directions

1. Preheat oven to 345 ºF.
2. Separate egg yolks from whites. Whisk the yolks to a pale yellow color. Add erythritol and stevia and mix until evenly combined.
3. Add fatty cream, coconut oil, and lemon juice.
4. Wash and zest the lemon. Add zest to the mixture and mix.
5. Add the coconut flour and baking powder. Mix all the ingredients.
6. Add the blackberry to the mixture. Press the berries into it a little. Bake pudding for 20-25 minutes.

Fat – 18g   Carbs – 4g   Protein -7g   Calories -158

WEEK 3

MEAL	Breakfast	Lunch	Snacks	Dinner	Dessert
Week 3					
SUNDAY	Keto Caesar Salad	Keto Paleo Scotch Eggs	Grilled Shrimp and Avocado	Braised Beef and Zucchini	Vegan Chocolate Orange Truffles
MONDAY	Keto Chicken Salad	Bacon Cheeseburger Soup	Coconut Oil Keto Bombs	Hearty Chicken Stew	Keto Chips with Zucchini
TUESDAY	Tuna, Greens, and Eggs Salad	Creamy Taco Soup (Low Carb)	Keto Easter «Cake»	Beef Stew	Festive Keto Terrine
WEDNESDAY	Tuna, Greens, and Eggs Salad	Wine-Coffee Beef Stew	Buffalo Deviled Eggs	Low Carb Pork Pie	Lemon Cheesecake
THURSDAY	Greek Salad	Keto Creamy Chicken Bacon Soup (instant pot)	Raspberry Lemon Ice Bombs	Green Chile Pork Stew	Keto Livers Truffles
FRIDAY	Keto Cheese Rolls	Stroganoff Soup Keto	Chocolate-Coconut Keto Candies	Venison Spring Keto Stew	Chocolate Keto Ice Cream
SATURDAY	Stuffed Cheese Bell Pepper	Japanese Clear Onion Soup	Keto bombs with Philadelphia Cream Cheese	Low Carb Pork Pie	Chocolate Coconut Fat Bombs

WEEK 3 SHOPPING LIST

PANTRY STAPLES	VEGETABLES
Butter	Avocados – 2 total
Cocoa powder -1 oz	Bell peppers – 12 oz
Coconut Milk – 2 pack	Lettuce - 16 oz
Coconut oil – 10 oz	Onions – 7 total
Canned tuna -4 can (16 oz)	Lemon – 5 total
Campari tomatoes – 3 lb	Cauliflower - ½ lb
	Spinach – 10 oz
DAIRY & MEAT	Olives –16 oz
Heavy Cream –10 oz	Zucchini – 4 total
Soft Cream Cheese – 8 containers (48 oz)	
Feta cheese – 8 oz	**OTHER**
Cheddar Cheese – 2 oz	Mushrooms –16 oz
Eggs – 30 total	Shrimp –1 lb
Bacon slices –25 oz	Champignons – 24 oz
Mascarpone – 5 oz	Dark chopped chocolate – 2 oz
Pork tenderloin –5 lb	
Chicken – 24 oz	
Chicken breast – 16 oz	
Chicken liver – 4 oz	
Mozzarella –8 oz	
Beef sirloin 2 lb	
Beef snack, tail -5 lb	
Sour cream – 24 oz	
Ground pork - 1 lb	
Parmesan cheese grated –10 oz	
Diced tomatoes – 5 oz	
Beef Stew –6 lb	
Venison – 1 lb	

DAY 15

Low calories day. Try to limit physical activity today.

Keto Caesar Salad
Keto Paleo Scotch Eggs
Grilled Shrimp and Avocado
Braised Beef and Zucchini
Vegan Chocolate Orange Truffles
Fat - 71g Carbs - 27g   Protein -100g Calories -1147

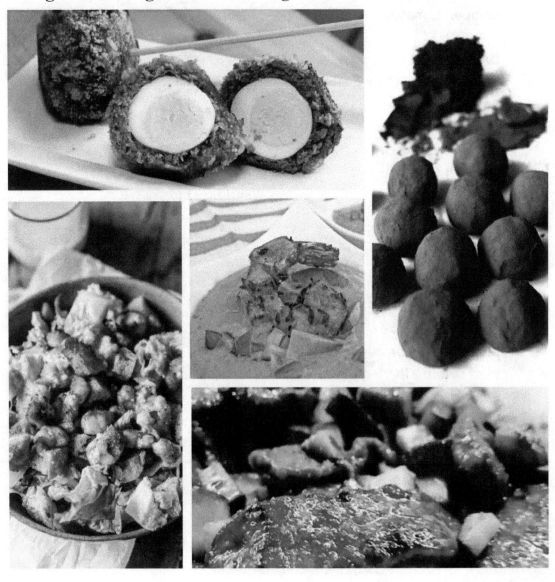

KETO CAESAR SALAD
4 serves | 30 min

Ingredients

2/3 pound chicken breasts

3 ounces bacon

½ pound Romaine lettuce

 2 ounces grated parmesan cheese

1 tablespoon olive oil

½ cup homemade mayonnaise

1 tablespoon Dijon mustard

½ lemon (juice)

2 tablespoons chopped anchovy filets

1 pressed garlic clove (to taste)

salt and pepper

Directions

Salad

1. Preheat the oven to 400 °F. Grease baking sheet. Place the chicken breasts on sheet.
2. Drizzle olive oil on top of the chicken. Add salt and pepper to breasts.
3. Bake the chicken for 20 minutes, until fully cooked.
4. Fry the bacon until crispy in the frying pan.
5. Shred the lettuce and place on plate.
6. Place sliced chicken on plate, crumble bacon on top.
7. Season the salad with dressing and 30 g grated Parmesan.

Dressing

Mix anchovies' filets, homemade mayonnaise, Dijon mustard, lemon juice, 2 tablespoons grated Parmesan cheese, garlic clove, salt and pepper with immersion blender. Chill in the refrigerator.

Fat – 32g   Carbs – 10g Protein -36g   Calories -468

Fat – 32g   Carbs – 10g Protein -36g   Calories -468

KETO PALEO SCOTCH EGGS

6 serves | 40 min

Ingredients

6 boiled eggs

1 pound mince pork, beef, or lamb

2 teaspoons herbs to taste

1 teaspoon onion flake salt

salt

Directions

1. Hard boil the eggs.
2. Mix minced meat, herbs and salt.
3. Cover the eggs with the meat completely. You can press the meat.
4. Preheat oven to 350 ºF.
5. Place the scotch eggs on the baking sheet. Brush them with oil. Sprinkle on onion flakes.
6. Bake the eggs for 15-20 minutes until golden all over.

Fat – 11g   Carbs – 1g   Protein -29g   Calories -219

GRILLED SHRIMP AND AVOCADO

9 serves | 15 min

Ingredients

1 pound shrimp (16 shrimp)

½ teaspoon salt

1 teaspoon black pepper

1 tablespoon onion powder

1 lemon

2 tablespoons coconut aminos

2 tablespoons avocado oil

2 ripe Hass avocados

Directions

1. Peel and clean the shrimp. Place them in a bowl.

2. Add salt, coconut aminos, pepper, onion powder. Add the juice of one half of the lemon. Combine.

3. Heat the grill or frying pan. Add avocado oil. Place shrimp in pan and cook for 3 minutes. Flip the shrimp.

4. Remove the shrimp and cool.

5. Peel and mush avocado with the fork. Add a little salt and lemon juice.

6. Put avocado mixture and the shrimp on the plate

Fat – 9g   Carbs – 4g   Protein -14g   Calories -152

BRAISED BEEF AND ZUCCHINI
4 serves | 55 min

Ingredients

2/3 pound beef

1/3 pound zucchini

1 onion

2 tablespoons butter

salt

pepper

Directions

1. Cut beef and onions into small pieces.
2. Put the butter in a frying pan, and add the beef and onions. Fry until golden brown on high heat.
3. Add a little water, cover and stew for one hour on low heat.
4. Cut the zucchini into slices. Add the vegetables and spices to the beef and stew for 30 minutes.

Fat – 18g   Carbs – 3g   Protein -20g   Calories -256

VEGAN CHOCOLATE ORANGE TRUFFLES

8 serves | 10 min

Ingredients

½ cup pitted dates

1 ounce almond meal

1 tablespoon unsweetened cocoa powder

Extra cocoa powder (for rolling the balls)

1 tablespoon orange juice

Zest of 1 lemon

Directions

1. Place pitted dates, almond meal, cocoa powder, orange juice, and lemon zest in a food processor or a powerful blender. Mix well.
2. Make the mixture into balls using your hands. Make 8 truffles.
3. Roll the candies in cocoa powder to taste.

Fat – 2g   Carbs – 10g   Protein -1g   Calories -52

DAY 16

Keto Chicken Salad
Bacon Cheeseburger Soup
Coconut Oil Keto Bombs
Hearty Chicken Stew
Keto Chips with Zucchini
Fat - 109g   Carbs - 30g   Protein -126g Calories -1573

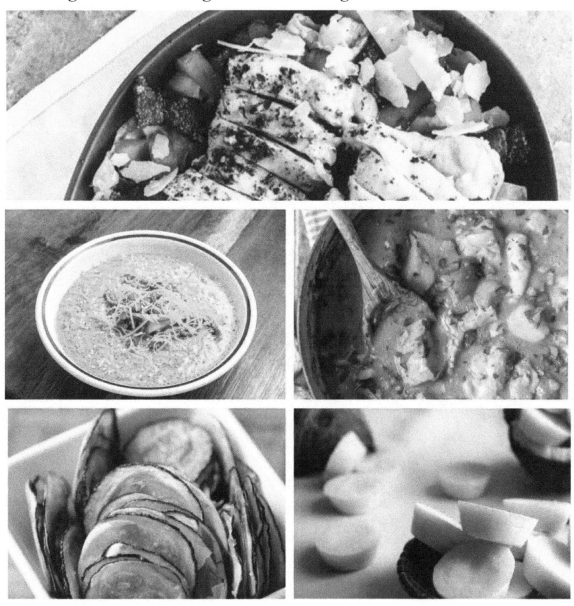

KETO CHICKEN SALAD

2 serves | 20 min

Ingredients

2/3 pound chicken breast

3 ounces thin-cut bacon slices

½ pound avocado

½ ounce mixed leaf greens

 2 ounces Paleo Ranch Dressing

Duck fat for greasing

Directions

1. Preheat the oven to 400 ºF.
2. Crisp the chicken breasts. Season with salt and pepper.
3. Grease pan with fat. Place breasts skin side down on the pan. Fry for 5-6 minutes. Flip the chicken and cook 30 seconds. Than transfer pan in the oven. Cook 10-15 minutes, until chicken is cooked through.
4. Place the slices bacon on the bake sheet. Bake the bacon slices in the oven until crispy. Alternatively, crisp the bacon in a frying pan.
5. Remove chicken from the oven. Cool for 5 minutes.
6. Slice the avocado and cooked chicken.
7. Place leafy greens on the plate. Add avocado, crispy bacon and sliced chicken.
8. Top with Ranch dressing.

Fat – 48g Carbs – 12g Protein -48g Calories -627

BACON CHEESEBURGER SOUP

6 serves | 40 min

Ingredients

5 slices bacon

2/3 pound ground beef

2 tablespoons butter

3 cups beef broth

½ teaspoon garlic powder

½ teaspoon onion powder

2 teaspoons yellow mustard

½ teaspoon black pepper

½ teaspoon ground red pepper

1 teaspoon cumin

1 teaspoon chili powder

2 ½ tablespoons tomato paste

3 medium diced dill pickle

1 cup shredded cheddar cheese

3 ounces cream cheese

½ cup heavy cream

Directions

1. Preheat the frying pan over medium heat. Place strips of bacon in it. Fry bacon for 5 minutes.
2. Remove bacon from the pan. Cook ground beef in the bacon grease for 10-15 minutes.
3. Take the other pan, preheat it. Place butter and spices in it. Cook for 45 seconds.
4. Add broth, mustard, tomato paste, cream cheese to the pan. Cook for 5 minutes, until cream cheese is melting.
5. Add pickles, heavy cream to the sauce, cook until of creamy brown texture.

6. Pour sauce over beef in a frying pan, and add bacon. Simmer for about 5-10 minutes.

Fat – 30g *Carbs – 5g* *Protein -32g* *Calories -419*

COCONUT OIL KETO BOMBS

10 serves | 10 min

Ingredients

4 ounces cream cheese

1/2 cup heavy cream, whipped

1 teaspoon orange vanilla

1/2 cup coconut oil

10 drops of liquid stevia

Directions

1. Mix all ingredients in a blender. Soften them in the microwave if it is difficult to mix the ingredients.
2. Freeze the mixture in silicone molds for 3–4 hours.
3. After freezing, remove the bombs from the molds and store in the refrigerator.

Fat – 19g   Carbs – 1g   Protein -1g   Calories -177

HEARTY CHICKEN STEW

6 serves | 45 min

Ingredients

6 chicken pieces (thighs and legs)

2 small zucchini, sliced into rounds

2 onions

4 medium carrots, peeled and sliced into rounds

2 cups white button mushrooms, halved

2 cups vegetable broth

1 teaspoon ground coriander

1 cup baby potatoes

1 teaspoon dried thyme

salt and pepper, to taste

Directions

1. Fry chicken, seasoned with thyme, coriander, salt, and pepper on a heated large pot until the skin has browned.
2. Mix all ingredients in the pot and bring it to a boil. Simmer for about 30 minutes, covered.

Fat – 11g   Carbs – 12g   Protein -44g   Calories -333

KETO CHIPS WITH ZUCCHINI

10 serves | 1 h 30 min

Ingredients

1 small zucchini, peeled, chopped

1 ounce sunflower seeds

1/2 teaspoons salt, or to taste

1/2 teaspoons paprika, or to taste

1/4 teaspoon turmeric, or to taste

1/4 teaspoon hot pepper flakes, or to taste

Directions

1. Put chopped zucchini and sunflower seeds into a blender.
2. Add spices to the mixture and blend.
3. Preheat the oven to 190°F.
4. Put the mixture on a baking sheet lined with parchment paper. Smooth it out to a thickness of about 1/4 inch.
5. Bake the zucchini mixture for 1–1 1/2 hours. If the chips are non-crunchy after that, bake for a little longer.
6. Remove from the oven and let cool a little before cutting or breaking into 10 chips. (A pizza cutter is ideal for this).

Fat – 1g   Carbs – 1g   Protein -1g   Calories -17

DAY 17

Tuna, Greens, and Eggs Salad
Creamy Taco Soup (Low Carb)
Keto Easter «Cake»
Beef Stew
Festive Keto Terrine
Fat - 86g Carbs - 29g   Protein -137g Calories -1622

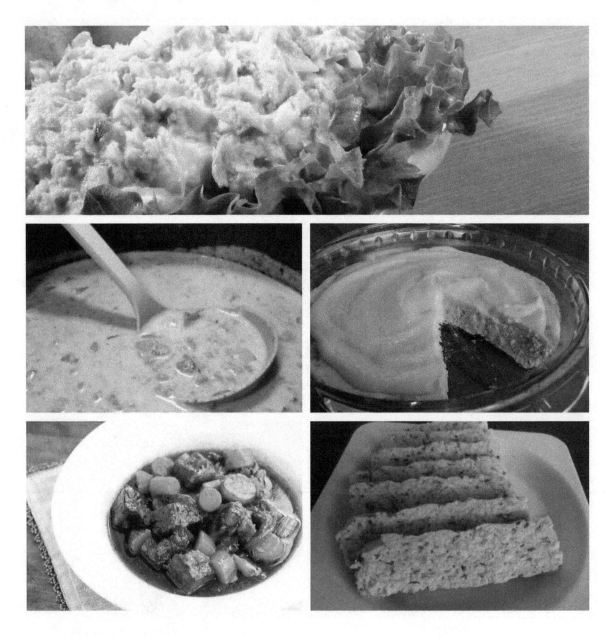

TUNA, GREENS, AND EGGS SALAD
4 serves | 30 min

Ingredients

1/3 pound canned tuna

¼ pound lettuce

2 chicken eggs

1 medium onion

2 tablespoons mayonnaise

lemon juice

salt

Directions

1. Cut the lettuce and put it on the plate.
2. Open the can and remove the tuna. Cut pieces, if necessary.
3. Mince the onion, and put it on the fish.
4. Boil the eggs. Cut them in half lengthwise.
5. Season the salad with mayo. Add a couple drops of lemon juice and salt.

Fat – 9g   Carbs – 5g   Protein -15g   Calories -167

CREAMY TACO SOUP (LOW CARB)
6 serves | 1 h 20 min

Ingredients

Soup:

2 teaspoons avocado oil (or butter)

1 onion

1 pound ground beef

2 tablespoons taco seasoning

1 14-ounce cans diced tomatoes

2 cups chicken broth

1/2 cup ranch dressing

1/3 pound cream cheese

Toppings:

1 ounce sliced olives

3 sliced green onions

2 ounces cilantro fresh (to taste)

1/2 avocado (optional)

1/2 cup cheddar cheese

1/2 cup sour cream

Directions

1. Take a small stock pot. Melt the butter in it over medium heat.
2. Peel and chop the onions, add to the pot. Stir onions occasionally until translucent.
3. Add ground beef and taco seasoning. Cook until ground beef is brown.
4. Add diced tomatoes.
5. Stir in broth, mix well. Simmer for about 20-30 minutes.
6. Add ranch dressing, cream cheese. Cook until cream cheese is melting, for 5 minutes.
7. Add salt and pepper to taste.

8.   After cooking, serve soup and garnish with cheddar cheese, chopped green onion, sour cream, cilantro, avocado, and olives.

Fat – 26g   Carbs – 11g   Protein -36g   Calories -575

KETO EASTER "CAKE"

1 serves | 30 min

Ingredients

9 ounces of soft cream cheese (such as Mascarpone)

7 ounces butter at room temperature

1 teaspoon sweetener (granulated stevia)

a pinch of vanilla

2 ounces of full-fat sour cream sweetened with 1 teaspoon sweetener (for example, stevia)

Directions

1. Mix cream cheese with butter adding sweetener, vanilla extract, and blueberries
2. Completely fill the mold (for the big cupcake) and refrigerate for at least two hours.
3. Turn the mold over and gently remove the "cake".
4. Serve with the sweetened sour cream.

Note: It is not a cottage cheese Easter cake, but it's very, very keto.

Fat – 16g   Carbs – 2g   Protein -3g   Calories -158

BEEF STEW
6 serves | 4 h

Ingredients

5 pounds beef snack, tail

3 medium carrots

8 Campari tomatoes

2 medium onions

2 ounces tomato sauce

8 cloves garlic

2 teaspoons garlic powder

2 tablespoons apple cider vinegar

2 cups chicken broth

2 cups water

2 teaspoons onion powder

4 teaspoons salt

3 teaspoons crushed red pepper

2 teaspoons parsley

1 teaspoon cayenne

2 teaspoons black pepper

2 teaspoons basil

3 whole bay leaves, spices, to taste

Directions

1. Pell and cut carrots, tomatoes, onion, garlic into chunky pieces.
2. Preheat the frying pan over medium heat.
3. Place vegetables and spices on the frying pan, stir and cook until translucent.
4. Replace the ingredients in the soup pot.
5. Take another cast iron skillet. Place beef snack in it. Cook on both sides, until crispy.

6. Pour broth into the pot to the onion, carrot and garlic.
7. Add two cups of water, apple cider vinegar. Cook for 2-3 minutes. Stir.
8. Add tomatoes, tomato sauce. Stir well.
9. Submerge beef tails into the broth. Boil the ingredients.
10. Reduce the heat to a simmer. Cover the pot.
11. Slightly simmer on a low heat for 3 hours.
12. When meat is cooked, it will be very soft and tender.
13. Remove the bay leaves from the pot. Serve.

Fat – 22g   Carbs – 9g   Protein -68g   Calories -531

FESTIVE KETO TERRINE
8 serves | 1 hour (+ 10 hours in the fridge)

Ingredients

5 ounces mascarpone cheese

2 ounces full-fat sour cream

1 pound skin-less, bone-less chicken breast fillets

5 ounces heavy cream

2 teaspoons gelatin

3 tablespoons hot water

1/2 teaspoons salt and pepper or to taste

1/2 tablespoons black sesame seeds

greens of your choice for serving

Directions

1. Cut chicken breast into cubes and boil them for 15 minutes.
2. Dissolve gelatin completely in the hot water and let it swell. Pour it into the sour cream.
3. Add salt and pepper to taste to the sour cream and gelatin.
4. Pour the mixture into a terrine mold.
   Place the mold in the fridge.
5. While the sour cream is cooling, whip the heavy cream with mascarpone cheese for about 1–2 minutes. Add salt and pepper.
6. Add chilled pieces of chicken and sesame seeds, and mix well.
7. When the gelatin-sour cream mixture has set, spoon the chicken mixture on top.
8. Place the dish in the fridge overnight.
9. In the morning remove the terrine from the mold by inverting it over a plate. If the mixture is stuck in the mold. Warm it slightly in warm water or with a hair dryer and run a knife around the side. Do not make it too warm.
10. Use a second plate and invert the terrine once more so the bottom of the terrine is now on the plate.
11. Sprinkle the terrine with finely chopped greens, cranberries orsome other garnish of your choice.

Fat – 13g   Carbs – 2g   Protein -15g   Calories -192

DAY 18

Tuna, Greens, and Eggs Salad
Wine-Coffee Beef Stew
Buffalo Deviled Eggs
Low Carb Pork Pie
Lemon Cheesecake
Fat - 92g Carbs - 17g   Protein -128g   Calories -1410

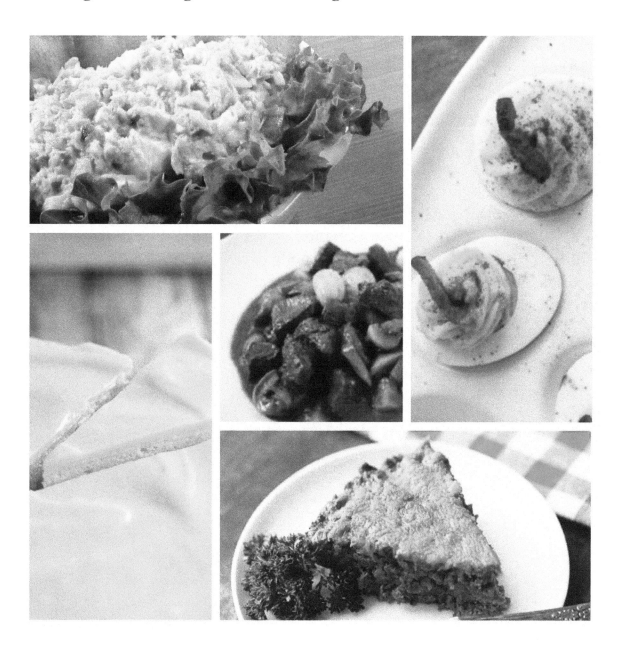

TUNA, GREENS, AND EGGS SALAD

4 serves | 30 min

Ingredients

1/3 pound canned tuna

¼ pound lettuce

2 eggs

1 medium onion

2 tablespoons mayonnaise

lemon juice

salt

Directions

1. Cut the lettuce and put it on the plate.
2. Open the can and remove the tuna. Cut pieces, if necessary.
3. Mince the onion, and put it on the fish.
4. Boil the eggs. Cut them in half lengthwise.
5. Season the salad with mayo. Add a couple drops of lemon juice and salt.

Fat – 9g   Carbs – 5g   Protein -15g   Calories -167

WINE-COFFEE BEEF STEW
6 serves | 3 h 30 min

Ingredients

3 pounds stew meat

3 cups coffee

1 cup beef stock

1 ½ cup baby bella mushrooms

2/3 cup red wine

1 medium onion

3 tablespoons coconut oil

2 tablespoons capers

2 teaspoons garlic

1 teaspoon salt

1 teaspoon pepper

Directions

1. Cut all stew meat in cubes.
2. Slice onions and mushrooms thinly.
3. Take a deep frying pan; pour 3 tablespoons coconut oil in it. Preheat the frying pan.
4. Place beef on the pan. Season beef with salt and pepper.
5. Fry meat in small batches. Place all meat in the pan after browning.
6. Place onion, mushrooms in the saucepan with the remaining fat. Cook until onion is translucent.
7. Pour coffee, beef stock, red wine, add capers to the vegetables and stir this mixture.
8. Add beef into the mixture, bring to a boil, and then reduce the heat to low.
9. Cover and cook for 3 hours.

Fat – 32g   Carbs – 3g   Protein -43g   Calories -504

BUFFALO DEVILED EGGS

6 serves | 30 min

Ingredients

6 hard boiled chicken eggs, large

1/3 pound boiled and chopped chicken

¼ onion

¼ cup blue cheese crumbles

¼ cup Franks Buffalo Wing Sauce

1 small chopped celery

2 tablespoons blue cheese dressing

Directions

1. Boil the eggs.
2. Chop the chicken and celery.
3. Peel cooked and cooled eggs. Cut them in half lengthwise. Separate the yolks from the egg whites and place yolks in mixing bowl.
4. Add chicken, celery, blue cheese, Franks Buffalo Wing Sauce and dressing to yolks.
5. Press the onion and add juice to the bowl. Mix all the ingredients.
6. Stuff the egg whites with yolk mixture using a fork or spoon. You can also pipe the yolks into the whites using a Ziploc bag with the tip cut off.

Fat – 12g   Carbs – 2g   Protein -29g   Calories -152

LOW CARB PORK PIE
4 serves | 1 h 15 min

Ingredients

1 pound ground pork

4 tablespoons grated Parmesan cheese

2 large eggs

½ lemon zest

½ teaspoon ground nutmeg

½ teaspoon ginger

½ teaspoon cardamom

4 tart shells

salt and pepper to taste

Directions

1. Heat a pan. Add meat and spices. Cook for 10-15 minutes over medium heat, and then remove a pan from heat. Add the eggs, cheese, and lemon zest.
2. Preheat the oven to 325 ºF.
3. Place mixture into pie shells. Bake for 20-25 minutes in oven.
4. Remove pie from the oven. Let cool and serve.

Fat – 12g   Carbs – 5g   Protein -36g   Calories -317

LEMON CHEESECAKE
4 serves | 10 min

Ingredients

½ pound soft cream cheese

2 ounces fatty cream

1 tablespoon lemon juice

1 teaspoon stevia in liquid form

1 teaspoon lemon peel

vanilla

Directions

1. Put cream cheese and cream on a bowl.
   Mix them with a mixer until uniform mass.
2. Add stevia, lemon juice, vanilla, lemon zest. Mix well.
3. Put the mixture into tart pans you may consume immediately. For best results, chill in the refrigerator for two hours to harden.

Fat – 27g   Carbs – 3g   Protein -6g   Calories -270

DAY 19

Low calories day. Try to limit physical activity today.

Greek Salad

Keto Creamy Chicken Bacon Soup (instant pot)

Raspberry Lemon Ice Bombs

Green Chile Pork Stew

Keto Livers Truffles

Fat - 132g   Carbs – 31g   Protein -121g Calories -1152

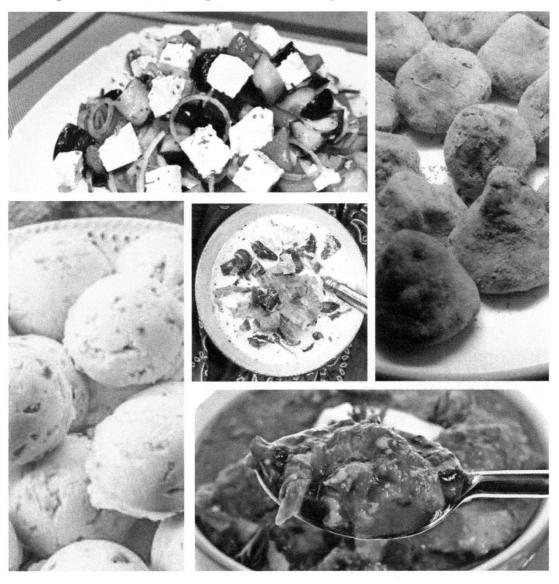

GREEK SALAD

4 serves | 15 min

Ingredients

2 ripe tomatoes

½ cucumber

½ red onion

½ green bell pepper

½ pound feta cheese

10 black olives

2 tablespoons olive oil

½ tablespoon red wine vinegar

2 teaspoons dried oregano

salt and pepper

Directions

Salad

1. Cut the tomatoes and cucumber into bite-sized pieces.
2. Thinly slice the bell pepper and onion.
3. Arrange the ingredients on a plate.
4. Add feta and olives.
5. Drizzle the salad with the dressing.
6. Sprinkle with oregano.

Dressing

Mix the olive oil and vinegar. Add salt and pepper to taste.

Fat – 20g   Carbs – 10g   Protein -9g   Calories -252

CREAMY CHICKEN BACON SOUP (INSTANT POT)

6 serves | 40 min

Ingredients

6 chicken thighs, boneless

½ pound cream cheese full fat

3 teaspoons minced garlic

1 cup frozen the chopped onion-celery mix

1/3 pound sliced mushrooms

4 teaspoons butter

1 teaspoon thyme

salt and pepper to taste

3 cups chicken broth

1 cup heavy cream

1 pound chopped cooked bacon

2 cups fresh spinach

Directions

1. Cut chicken thighs into cubes, place into a large zipper bag.
2. Add full-fat cream cheese, minced garlic, frozen chopped onion-celery mix, sliced mushrooms, butter, thyme, salt, and pepper to taste to the zipper bag. Place the bag in a fridge.
3. At the same time pour chicken mixture into Instant Pot.
4. Add chicken broth and cook for 30 minutes. Use the soup setting.
5. Mix well the ingredients, add spinach and cream.
6. Cover the instant pot and let it sit for 10 minutes until spinach wilt.
7. At the same time slice and cut the bacon. Place the slices in the frying pan. Cook for 5 minutes.
8. Pour the soup in a bowl and top with fried bacon.

Fat – 63g   Carbs – 7g   Protein -77g   Calories -452

RASPBERRY LEMON ICE BOMBS
6 serves | 2 h 30 min

Ingredients

1/4 cup coconut oil

1 cup coconut milk

1/4 cup sour cream

1/4 cup cream

3 1/2 ounces raspberries

juice of half a lemon

20 drops liquid stevia

Directions

1. Put all the ingredients in a blender and blend until the raspberries mix with the rest of the products.
2. Strain the mixture to remove the raspberry seeds. It's important because the seeds in the finished ice bombs will irritate the tongue.
3. Pour the mixture into 5 silicone molds and freeze for two hours.

Fat – 25g   Carbs – 6g   Protein -2g   Calories -246

GREEN CHILE PORK STEW
8 serves | 1 h 45 min

Ingredients

2 pounds pork loin

2 teaspoons ground cumin

2 teaspoons granulated garlic

1 teaspoon pure ground chile powder (to taste)

2 ounces chopped onion

2 cloves garlic

3 cups whole hatch green chilies and liquid

3 tablespoons oil

2 cups water

poached eggs optional

salt to taste

Directions

1. Cut pork loin into cubes.
2. Preheat oil in a big frying pan. Fry pork until brown.
3. Add spices to the pork. Cook until fragrant.
4. At the same time chop garlic and onion. Place ingredients in a food processor.
5. Add canned chilies to the food processor. Mix and make thick chunky paste.
6. Add chili and onion mixture to the pork. Pour the liquid of canned chilies.
7. Pour two cups of water.
8. Stir the ingredients and make low-heat. Cover the pan with a lid.
9. Simmer the stew for 60-90 minutes until pork is tender.
10. Add a little water during the last hour cooking.
11. Before finishing, add salt to taste.
12. Serve stew with the poached eggs.

Fat – 10g   Carbs – 4g   Protein -20g   Calories -182

KETO LIVERS TRUFFLES
12 serves | 50 min

Ingredients

3 ounces soft cheese

7 ounces chicken livers

1 teaspoon butter

1 tablespoon cognac

1–2 tablespoons cocoa powder

1–2 tablespoons mixture of seeds (chia, sesame, flax seed)

olive oil, salt, pepper

Directions

1. Preheat a frying pan. Cook the livers in olive oil for 5 minutes on high heat. Add cognac and flame it or you can just let it evaporate. Reduce the heat, add the butter and continue cooking the livers until done. Remove the livers from the pan and allow them to cool.
2. Mix cold livers with the cheese in a food processor. Put liver-cheese mix in the fridge before forming truffles.
3. Make 12 balls from liver-cheese mixture (wet hands will be better). Roll some balls into the cocoa and some into the mixture of seeds. Serve.

Note: If you are having a buffet, serve the truffles in a small paper basket as for homemade chocolates.

Fat – 2g   Carbs – 1g   Protein -5g   Calories -40

DAY 20

Keto Cheese Rolls

Stroganoff Soup Keto

Chocolate-Coconut Keto Candies

Venison Spring Keto Stew

Chocolate Keto Ice Cream

Fat - 100g   Carbs - 31g   Protein -98g   Calories -1420

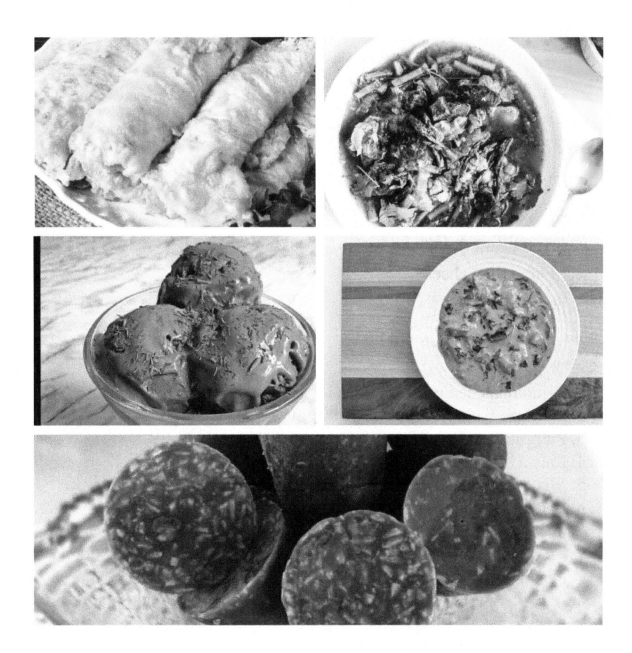

KETO CHEESE ROLLS
3 serves | 30 min

Ingredients

4 eggs, separated

1 clove of garlic, peeled and crushed

2 ounces hard cheese, grated

4 tablespoons homemade mayonnaise

3 ounces cauliflower (can be frozen), blanched

2 pieces of melted cheese

black pepper to taste

1 bunch greens to taste, chop finely

Directions

1. Grind blanched cauliflower in a blender or grinder for 5 minutes.
2. Beat egg whites into a creamy foam and set aside.
3. Preheat oven to 350°F.
4. Line a baking sheet with parchment paper.
5. Mix cauliflower with yolks, and then gently fold in the whites.
6. Put the mixture on the baking sheet and smooth it out. Place it in the oven for 15 minutes.
7. Mix the grated cheese with garlic, spices, salt, greens and homemade mayonnaise for the toppings.
8. After baking, remove the base from the oven. Place the toppings on it and spread it over the base. Take one edge of the base and gently roll it like a jelly-roll. Lay it on a plate and slice the roll into 3 portions.

Fat – 20g   Carbs – 9g   Protein -15g   Calories -269

STROGANOFF HIGH FAT SOUP

6 serves | 1 h

Ingredients

2 pounds Sirloin Beef

1 ½ pound Champignon

2 ounces Ghee

2 cloves minced garlic

¼ pound medium chopped white onion

5 cups bone, chicken or vegetable broth

2 teaspoons paprika

1 tablespoon Dijon mustard

4 tablespoons lemon juice

2/3 pound sour cream

1/4 cup freshly chopped parsley

1 teaspoon salt

1/4 teaspoon freshly ground black pepper

Directions

1. Slice beef into thin strips. Season with some salt and pepper.
2. Clean and slice the mushrooms.
3. Grease a large, heavy bottom pan with half of the ghee. Preheat the pan. Try to add beef in one layer. Fry slices over medium-high heat quickly until the meat becomes brown on all sides. Repeat for the remaining slices.
4. Remove slices from the pan, place them in a bowl. Set aside.
5. Grease a pan with the remaining ghee. Place chopped onion and minced garlic in the pan. Cook for about 2-3 minutes.
6. Add sliced mushrooms to the pan. Cook for 3-5 minutes.
7. Add Dijon mustard, paprika. Mix the ingredients. Pour bone broth in a pan.
8. Add lemon juice and bring to a boil. Cook for 2-3 minutes.

9. Add the browned beef slices and sour cream. Cook for 1-2 minutes, take off the heat.

Fat – 31g   Carbs – 7g   Protein -47g   Calories -520

CHOCOLATE-COCONUT KETO CANDIES

20 serves | 1 h 5 min

Ingredients

2 ounces butter, melted

2 tablespoons coconut flakes

1/2 ounce of any nuts, crushed

1/2 tablespoon cocoa powder

1 teaspoon granulated sweetener to taste

1 teaspoon vanilla extract

Directions

1. Melt the butter. Mix all ingredients and add them to the melted butter. Stir well.

2. Use a small rectangular mold. Pour the mixture into it. Put the mold into the refrigerator for 1–4 hours.

3. When it is hard, remove it from the refrigerator and cut the hard mass into 20 pieces of candy.

Note: should keep refrigerated.

Fat – 6g Carbs – 1g   *Protein -0g*   *Calories -54*

VENISON SPRING HFLC STEW

4 serves | 4 h 20 min

Ingredients

1 pound venison

2 tablespoons olive oil

1 bulb garlic

1 cup shredded cabbage (purple)

1 cup sliced celery

4 cups bone broth

1 teaspoon salt

1 teaspoon pepper

2 cups chopped asparagus

2 bay leaves

Directions

1. At first, peel and slice garlic. Cut it into 1/8-inch thin slices.
2. Slice the purple cabbage.
3. Slice celery.
4. Preheat the skillet. Pour olive oil in it.
5. Add celery, garlic, bay leaves to the skillet. Saute the ingredients for about 5-6 minutes until tender.
6. Add venison to the cabbage. Salt and pepper. Cook until the meat is brown.
7. Take a big saucepan. Place cabbage and venison in it, add broth.
8. Stew for 4 hours. Add water if the stew is dry.
9. When done, add chopped asparagus in the saucepan.
10. Serve the stew with olive oil and lime.

Fat – 16g   Carbs – 8g   Protein -32g   Calories -310

CHOCOLATE KETO ICE CREAM
6 serves | 3 h 20 min

Ingredients

2 ½ ounces coconut cream

2 ounces butter or coconut oil

1 tablespoon cocoa

1 teaspoon vanilla extract

1 2/3 cups coconut milk

1–2 teaspoons liquid sweetener

4 egg yolks

1/8 teaspoon xanthan gum (optional)

Directions

1. Whisk the egg yolks.
2. On low heat warm 1/2 cup of coconut milk with the vanilla extract in a small saucepan.
3. Stir vanilla milk and pour it slowly in a thin stream into the yolks, stirring gently. Do this gradually so that the eggs yolks do not coagulate. Cook the yolk mixture on low heat, stirring, for 5–7 minutes until the mix thickens. Don't let it boil. After that, cool the mixture down.
4. If you use xanthan gum, mix it with the liquid sweetener.
5. Slowly pour the sweetener into the beaten cold milk mixture, stirring. If you prefer not to use the xanthan gum, you can pour all the sweetener at once into the milk.
6. 6. Then gently mix the coconut milk-yolk mixture with the cocoa, butter or oil, and the coconut cream. Beat all ingredients together for 1–2 minutes.
7. You can use an ice cream maker for freezing the mixture.
8. Put the ice cream into the freezer for about 3–4 hours.

Note: This keto ice cream is for those who do not eat dairy products but, at the same time, love ice cream.

Fat – 27g   *Carbs – 6g*   *Protein -3g*   *Calories -267*

DAY 21

Low calories day. Try to limit physical activity today.

Stuffed Cheese Bell Pepper

Japanese Clear Onion Soup

Keto Bombs with Philadelphia Cream Cheese

Low Carb Pork Pie

Chocolate Coconut Fat Bombs

Fat - 46g Carbs - 31g   Protein -55g   Calories -1091

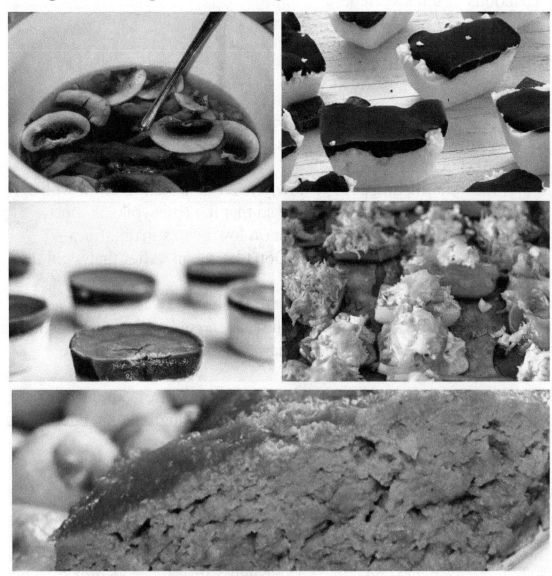

STUFFED CHEESE BELL PEPPER
4 serves | 45 min

Ingredients

2 bell peppers, 2/3 pound

2 eggs

½ cup Mozzarella cheese

½ cup Parmesan cheese

½ cup Ricotta cheese

3 tablespoons dried parsley

1 cup spinach

Salt

Directions

1. Preheat the oven to 370 ºF.
2. Wash and peel the peppers. Cut them in half lengthwise.
3. Mix cheese, eggs, and dried parsley in a blender.
4. Stuff each half with cheese mixture.
5. Put spinach on the top of the pepper. Bake for 30 min.
6. Sprinkle the Parmesan on the peppers and return to the oven for 5 min.

Fat – 9g   Carbs – 10g   Protein -15g   Calories -169

JAPANESE CLEAR ONION SOUP

4 serves | 40 min

Ingredients

2 onions, diced

6 cups water or vegetable broth

2 celery stalks, diced

2 carrots, diced

2 cloves of garlic

2 ounces button mushrooms, sliced

2 ounces scallions

1 tablespoon olive oil

salt, pepper, soy sauce, Sriracha sauce, to taste

Directions

1. Preheat the oil in a saucepan. Place onions in it. Saute the onions until slightly brown.
2. Add peeled and chopped carrots, onions, celery, garlic.
3. Pour 6 cups of water or broth.
4. Boil for 30 minutes.
5. Strain vegetables from the broth.
6. Peel and slice the mushrooms.
7. Cut scallions.
8. Add mushrooms, scallions to the broth before serving.
9. Add soy sauce, Sriracha to taste

Fat – 4g Carbs – 10g Protein -2g   Calories -100

KETO BOMBS WITH PHILADELPHIA CREAM CHEESE

8 serves | 40 min

Ingredients

For the bombs:

5 1/2 ounces Philadelphia cream cheese

2 ounces butter

2 ounces coconut oil

1/2 teaspoon erythritol

To taste granulated or liquid stevia sweetener

Vanilla extract or vanilla pods

For keto chocolate topping:

1 ounce cocoa powder

1 tablespoon coconut oil or cocoa butter

Stevia extract

Directions

1. Mix all the ingredients for the bombs together in a food processor until there is a uniform mixture.
2. Add the erythritol gradually, tasting from time to time for sweetness to your taste. You will need about 1/2 teaspoon of erythritol and one drop of stevia. Stir until it is completely dissolved.
3. Using small silicone or muffin molds, transfer the mixture to the molds. Fill them 3/4 full.
4. Place the bombs into the freezer for 15–20 minutes.
5. Meanwhile, prepare the keto chocolate topping. Heat grated cocoa with coconut oil in a water bath. Add only stevia extract for sweetness! Stir. When the mixture becomes well combined, remove from the heat and let cool slightly.
6. Remove the keto bombs from the freezer and pour chocolate mixture on them. Refrigerate for 2 more hours.

Fat – 2g   Carbs – 3g   Protein -1g   Calories -318

LOW CARB PORK PIE

4 serves | 1 h 15 min

Ingredients

1 pound ground pork

4 tablespoons grated Parmesan cheese

2 large eggs

½ lemon zest

½-teaspoon ground nutmeg

½-teaspoon ginger

½-teaspoon cardamom

4 tart shells

salt and pepper to taste

Directions

1. Heat a pan. Add meat and spices. Cook for 10-15 minutes over medium heat, and then remove a pan from heat. Add the eggs, cheese, and lemon zest.
2. Preheat the oven to 325ºF.
3. Place mixture into pie shells. Bake for 20-25 minutes in oven.
4. Remove pie from the oven. Let cool and serve.

Fat – 12g Carbs – 5g   Protein -36g   Calories -317

CHOCOLATE COCONUT FAT BOMBS

8 serves | 12 min

Ingredients

1/4 cup savory coconut flakes

1/4 cup liquid coconut oil

2 tablespoons erythritol

1/4 cup solid coconut oil

1 ounce dark chocolate (sugar-free, 85% or more cocoa content)

Directions

1. Melt the mixture of coconut oils in the microwave for 45 seconds to 1 minute and mix well.
2. Add coconut flakes and sweetener, and mix well again.
3. Pour the mixture into ice trays (or silicon molds) and freeze for 30 minutes.
4. Melt dark chocolate in the microwave for 1 minute.
5. Pour equally over each coconut bomb by the spoonfuls of chocolate.

Fat – 19g Carbs – 3g   Protein -1g   Calories -187

HIGH FAT LOW CARB FOOD LIST

All values are approximate from Google data, sorted from lowest to highest net carb count.

MEATS

ITEM / WEIGHT	NET CARBS
Bacon (1 Pan fried slice, 10g)	0
Beef (70/30 Ground, 100g)	0
Beef (85/15 Ground, 100g)	0
Beef (Brisket, 100g)	0
Chicken (Breast, 100g)	0
Chicken (Thighs, 100g)	0
Chicken (Drumsticks, 100g)	0
Chicken (Wings, 100g)	0
Crab (King, 100g)	0
Fish (Tuna, 100g)	0
Fish (Tilapia, 100g)	0
Fish (Salmon, 100g)	0
Fish (Catfish, 100g)	0
Fish (Halibut, 100g)	0
Fish (Sole, 85g)	0
Fish (Pacific Cod, 100g)	0
Fish (Pompano, 100g)	0
Lobster (cooked, 100g)	0
Pork (varies, 100g)	0
Turkey (Breast, 100g)	0
Turkey (Leg, 100g)	0
Turkey (Dark Meat, 100g)	0
Shrimp (85g)	0.2
Egg (Large, 50g)	0.6
Chicken (Liver, 100g)	1
Scallops (steamed, 100g)	5

HERBS & SPICES

ITEM / WEIGHT	NET CARBS
Cilantro (20g)	0.1
Thyme (0.8g)	0.1
Dill (1g)	0.1
Oregano (2g, ground, dried)	0.4

VEGETABLES

ITEM / WEIGHT	NET CARBS
Collard Greens (100g)	1
Lettuce (Romaine, 100g)	1
Bok Choy (100g)	1.2
Spinach (100g)	1.4
Lettuce (Green Leaf, 100g)	1.6
Celery (100g)	1.7
Asparagus (100g)	1.8
Radishes (100g)	1.8
Avocado (100g)	2
Cabbage (Napa, 100g)	2
Arugula (100g)	2.1
Mushrooms (White, 100g)	2.3
Yellow Squash (100g)	2.3
Zucchini (100g)	2.4
Mushrooms (Portobello, 100g)	2.6
Tomato (Red, 100g)	2.7
Olives (100g)	2.8
Bell Pepper (Green, 100g)	2.9
Eggplant (100g)	3
Cauliflower (100g)	3
Cucumbers (100g)	3.1
Cabbage (Green, 100g)	3.3
Green Beans (100g)	3.4
Bell Pepper (Red, 100g)	3.9
Kale (Boiled, 100g)	4
Jalapeno (100g)	4
Broccoli (100g)	4
Green Onions (100g)	4.6
Cabbage (Red, 100g)	4.6
Edamame (100g)	5
Bell Pepper (Yellow, 100g)	5
Brussel Sprouts (100g)	5.2
Spaghetti Squash (100g)	5.5
Artichokes (100g)	6

DAIRY

ITEM / WEIGHT	NET CARBS
Pepper Jack (28g / 1oz)	0
Monterey Jack (28g / 1oz)	0
Butter (1 tbsp)	0
Butter, Whipped (1 tbsp)	0
Cheddar (28g / 1oz)	0.4
Heavy Cream (1 tbsp)	0.4
Mozarella (28g / 1oz, Whole Milk)	0.6
Blue Cheese (28g / 1oz)	0.7
Mozarella (28g / 1oz, Skim Milk)	0.9
Half & Half (2 tbsp)	1
Parmesan (28g / 1oz)	1.2
Feta (28g / 1oz)	1.2
Cream Cheese (28g / 1oz)	1.5
Swiss (28g / 1oz)	1.5
Ricotta Cheese (100g)	3
Cottage Cheese (100g)	3.4

NOTES